The
Cholesterol Myths

Myth: Some scholars hold that in ancient religions the myth took the place of dogma. Myths not only have a religious purpose, but also an explanatory, or etiological one; e.g., they may offer interpretations of natural phenomena, or may explain established beliefs or customs.

The Columbia Encyclopedia

The
Cholesterol Myths

EXPOSING THE FALLACY
THAT CHOLESTEROL AND SATURATED FAT
CAUSE HEART DISEASE

Uffe Ravnskov, MD, PhD

Foreword by Michael Gurr, PhD

NewTrends Publishing, Inc.
Washington, DC

The Cholesterol Myths is intended solely for informational and educational purposes and not as personal medical advice. Please consult your doctor if you have any questions about your health— but it may also be a good idea for him or her to read this book.

The Cholesterol Myths:
Exposing the Fallacy
That Cholesterol and Saturated Fat
Cause Heart Disease

Cover and Book Design: Sally Fallon
23R-methyl substituted methyl ether derivative of cholesterol structure
    courtesy of Indiana University Molecular Structure Project

Library of Congress Cataloging-in-Publication Data

Ravnskov, Uffe
        The cholesterol myths: exposing the fallacy that
            cholesterol and saturated fat cause heart disease
        Uffe Ravnskov, MD, PhD; Foreword by Michael Gurr, PhD
            p.   cm.
        Includes bibliographical references and index
        ISBN   0-9670897-0-0
            1. Cholesterol   2. Coronary Heart Disease
            3. Atherosclerosis 4. Scientific Method
            5. Lipid Disorders   6. Diet
            7. Clinical Trials 8. Lipoproteins

Library of Congress Card Number: 00-107620
Printed in the United States of America
Printings: September 2000, 5000; March 2002, 10,000; March 2003, 10,000,

Published by NewTrends Publishing, Inc., Washington, DC
www.NewTrendsPublishing.com   newtrends@kconline.com
US and Canadian Orders (877) 707-1776
International Orders (574) 268-2601
Available to the trade through Biblio Distribution
(a division of NBN) 800-462-6420

To Bodil

Contents

Figures and Tables

Text Boxes

Illustrations

Foreword

by Michael Gurr, PhD

Whether diet plays a major role in heart disease is a question that interests us all. Author Ravnskov has a mission: To inform his readers that there is a side to this question other than the view usually presented to us.

Governments and health authorities never tire of reminding those of us who live in industrialized countries that heart disease is a major cause of death. They go further and tell us that heart disease is eminently preventable. While conceding that genetic background interacts with numerous environmental factors to influence each individual's risk of succumbing to heart attack, they insist that diet is foremost among these factors as a *cause* of heart disease, and that modifying diet provides a straightforward means of preventing heart attacks. If only people would do what they are advised—reduce their intake of fats, especially those rich in the saturated fatty acids—then the high toll of death and disability from this disease could be readily reduced. If only!

What is the scientific basis on which this advice is based? Although the many reports of "expert committees" acknowledge that diet may influence the underlying pathology of heart disease in several ways, current "dietary guidelines" are based mainly on what Dr. Ravnskov calls "the diet-heart idea." Greatly simplified (which it normally is!), this idea proposes that dietary fats rich in saturated fatty acids raise the concentration of cholesterol in the blood. This in turn is involved in the initiation of arteriosclerosis, which through its restriction of blood flow to the myocardium and its tendency to generate thrombi, leads to myocardial infarction.

Dr. Ravnskov's contention is that the diet-heart idea is a house built on sand. He leads us through the history of the concept in an interesting and readable way. His writing clearly demonstrates the enormous depth and range of his reading on this subject. Step by step he examines the evidence for the diet-heart idea, and step by step he shows us how that evidence may be flawed or contradicted by other research that is rarely acknowledged or quoted.

Medical science has generally been highly regarded by the public, who have rarely questioned its findings because it is perceived as helping to improve mankind's lot. It will come as a surprise to many readers to learn how many studies of diet and heart disease were poorly designed and conducted, how many did not produce the results that have been claimed for them and have been quoted irrelevantly or misleadingly, and how many published studies exist whose results seriously question or contradict the diet-heart idea but are never acknowledged or quoted. Some of these tactics are not only just misleading but also sometimes amount to scientific fraud.

Dr. Ravnskov is well qualified to write such a book. He is a general practitioner who regularly needs to advise patients who have heart disease or who are worried that they might have it. The book begins with an insight into problems of one such patient, an otherwise healthy woman who began to worry after a company health screen revealed that she had high cholesterol and who was told by the company medical officer that she might have a heart attack in five years if she didn't do anything. Dr. Ravnskov and many like him are concerned that public health messages based on poor science may not only be ineffective but also may cause unnecessary worry to people who were previously free of health cares.

As well as conducting his medical practice, Dr. Ravnskov is also a scientist who has published a number of papers, including some penetrating analyses of the diet-heart literature. He is one of a growing number of scientists who have found what they have read disconcerting.

Why do we hear so little about this alternative view? Few scientists seem willing to stand up and question what has become accepted dogma. Dr. Ravnskov lists a few at the end of his book and outlines their views and credentials. Most are, like the author, individuals with enquiring minds who are not directly involved in heart disease research. Some, however, have been eminent researchers into heart disease; their firm stand against conventional views has often alienated them from the establishment community. By contrast, many who support the consensus view have made their reputations in this field, have been supported by research grants often amounting to millions of dollars and have a vested interest in continuing to support and sustain the diet-heart idea.

Another dimension to this story that Dr. Ravnskov discusses is the approach to lowering cholesterol by drugs, which has almost always been more effective than diet. The cholesterol story, therefore, has the backing of the multimillion-dollar drug industry. While this backing is not reprehensible in itself, the distinction between the ability of drug and dietary treatment to lower blood cholesterol has often become so blurred that lay people are frequently confused into believing that dietary modification could achieve exactly the same effect as a drug treatment when it clearly cannot. Alternatively, many may be persuaded that they need drugs when clearly they do not.

Quite apart from showing us the flimsiness of the scientific evidence upon which dietary advice to prevent or reduce heart disease is based, Dr. Ravnskov also addresses an even more serious problem. Could attempts to reduce cardiovascular mortality by lowering blood cholesterol actually do harm? Several authors have reflected that it might and have cited the evidence. To this end, Ravnskov discusses the worrying observation that even when cardiovascular deaths have been reduced in some intervention trials, subjects died of other causes—sometimes cancer, sometimes suicide or other forms of violence—resulting in no overall change in death rate. Many "expert" committees reviewing this evidence have tended either to ignore this phenomenon or have argued that it can safely be disregarded, but the admonition "do no harm" comes back to haunt us.

Many with establishment views will regard Dr. Ravnskov as a crank. That would be a grave mistake. He has done his homework, he is not a lone voice in the wilderness, and he deserves to be taken seriously. Above all, this book will make us all think more deeply about the true role of diet in heart disease and about the quality of the information that we receive.

Michael Gurr, PhD
Visiting Professor in Food Science & Technology
University of Reading, Reading, UK

Visiting Professor in Human Nutrition
Oxford Brookes University, Oxford, UK

St. Mary's, January 1996

Author's Foreword

When the cholesterol campaign was introduced in Sweden in 1989, I was very surprised. Having followed the scientific literature about cholesterol and cardiovascular disease superficially for a number of years, I could not recall any study showing that high cholesterol was dangerous to the heart or the blood vessels, or that any type of dietary fat was more beneficial or harmful than another one. I became curious and started to read more systematically.

Anyone who reads the literature in this field with an open mind soon discovers that the emperor has no clothes, and so did I. I also soon learned that the critical analyses or comments that I sent to various medical journals were of little interest to the editors. The reviewers sent me mocking answers. Besides, the inaccuracies, misinterpretations, exaggerations and misleading quotations in this research area were so numerous that to question them all demanded a book.

The first edition of *The Cholesterol Myths* was published in Sweden in 1991 and in Finland in 1992. The books made little impact. In Sweden, the science journalists usually lost interest in the subject when, after reading the book, they consulted the researchers or the health authorities I had criticized. In Finland, the book was the subject of a television program on Channel 2 where it was belittled by some of the Finnish proponents and then—literally—set on fire!

The indiscriminate acceptance of the cholesterol campaign in Sweden was most probably due to its promotion by large American health and research institutions, such as the National Heart, Lung and Blood Institute and the American Heart Association, along with their influential members. Evidently, the Swedish health authorities must have thought that such prestigious authorities could not be wrong. But Sweden and Finland are small countries. I thought that perhaps I could reach more discerning and independent journalists and researchers by publishing the book in English. Many queries to publishers and literary agents were rejected, however; the book was considered of no commercial interest.

With the advent of the internet, I saw a way to inform the public, and in 1997 I published selected sections of the book on the web. According to the search engine Direct Hit, my website soon became one of the top ten most popular sites about cholesterol, and from email letters I learned that many laymen and researchers were just as skeptical about the cholesterol campaign and the diet-heart idea as I was—or at least they became skeptical after having read my website.

One of the correspondents was Sally Fallon, author of *Nourishing Traditions*. She had encountered the same problems in finding a publisher for her book, with its controversial emphasis on foods like butter and cream, and eventually set up her own publishing company to take the book to press. She asked whether she might publish *The Cholesterol Myths*.

All researchers stand on the shoulders of their predecessors, and so do I. Hopefully, I have paid credit to all of them in the book. But there are other important individuals who have contributed to this book in some way or another. First of all I would like to thank Bodil Jönsson and Olof Holmqvist for their many ingenious comments on the first draft. I am also greatly indebted to Linda Newman for her tremendous and unselfish work changing my first, broken translation of the Swedish edition into good English. At a later stage, when I had undone some of Linda's good work by updating and revising the text, Sally Fallon repaired the damage.

I would also like to mention here Lars Werkö, a critical researcher himself, who has given me invaluable support and encouragement throughout the years.

The following individuals have been important in various ways, either by giving me valuable, critical comments to the various drafts or simply by showing me their qualified appreciation of my work. This list includes, in alphabetical order, Poul Astrup, Jonas Bergström, Christer Enkvist, Michael Gurr, Joel Kauffmann, George Mann, James McCormick, Peter Nilsson-Ehle, Robert E. Olson, Eskil Richardson, Ray Rosenman, Kari Salminen, the late Petr Skrabanek, Lars Söderhjelm and Nicolai Worm.

Last, but certainly not least, this book would never have been written without the patience and encouragement of my wife, Bodil.

Uffe Ravnskov, MD, PhD
Lund, Sweden

Introduction

The Diet-Heart Idea: A Die-Hard Hypothesis

The great tragedy of Science—the slaying of a beautiful hypothesis by an ugly fact.

Thomas Huxley (1825-1895)

Did you know. . .

. . . that cholesterol is not a deadly poison, but a substance vital to the cells of all mammals?

. . . that your body produces three to four times more cholesterol than you eat?

. . . that this production increases when you eat only small amounts of cholesterol and decreases when you eat large amounts?

. . . that the "prudent" diet, low in saturated fat and cholesterol, cannot lower your cholesterol more than a small percentage?

. . . that the only effective way to lower cholesterol is with drugs?

. . . that many of the cholesterol-lowering drugs are dangerous to your health and may shorten your life?

. . . that the new cholesterol-lowering drugs, called statins, do lower heart-disease mortality, but this is because of effects other than cholesterol lowering? Unfortunately, they also stimulate cancer, at least in rodents.

. . . that you may become aggressive or suicidal if you lower your cholesterol too much?

. . . that polyunsaturated fatty acids, those which are claimed to prevent heart attacks, stimulate infections and cancer in rats?

. . . that if you eat too much polyunsaturated oil you will age faster than normal? You will see this on the outside as wrinkled skin. You can't see the effects of premature aging on the inside of your body, but you will certainly feel them.

. . . that too much polyunsaturated oil may provoke athero-sclerosis?

. . . that people whose blood cholesterol is low develop just as many plaques in their blood vessels as people whose choles-terol is high?

. . . that more than thirty studies of more than 150,000 individuals have shown that people who have had a heart attack haven't eaten more saturated fat or less polyunsaturated oil than other people?

. . . that old women with high cholesterol live longer than old women with low cholesterol?

. . . that many of these facts have been presented in scien-tific journals and books for decades but proponents of the diet-heart hypothesis never tell them to the public?

. . . that the diet-heart idea and the cholesterol campaign create immense prosperity for researchers, doctors, drug pro-ducers and the food industry?

A sorry story

Karla didn't know it.

Karla and I live in the southern part of Sweden, a prosper-ous country where nobody needs to starve. If anything, overweight is a problem for many people because good food is abundant.

In Sweden people grow old; the people of Sweden enjoy one of the longest life spans in the world. Therefore, heart failure is a common cause of death simply because heart failure is a disease of old age. But man is never satisfied, and great efforts are made to prolong life. One of these efforts is to determine which people have high cholesterol because scientists say that lowering cholesterol may prevent heart disease and give you a longer life. When you have read this book you will know that nothing could be more wrong. But first let me tell a little more about Karla.

Karla has been my patient for several years. On her occasional visits, she had always been cheerful and optimistic.

Now she is tired and depressed, not at all the way she used to be.

Karla is sixty-two. She works as a cleaner in the offices of a large factory. Two years ago the doctor at the company called all employees in for a medical checkup.

"Your cholesterol is too high," he told her. "There is a great risk that you will have a heart attack within five years if you don't do anything about it."

"I felt fit as a fiddle, but he scared me to death," Karla told me.

She doesn't feel fit any longer.

Karla was sent to the medical clinic at the nearest hospital where the doctor told her to go on a diet. Karla loves to eat and to

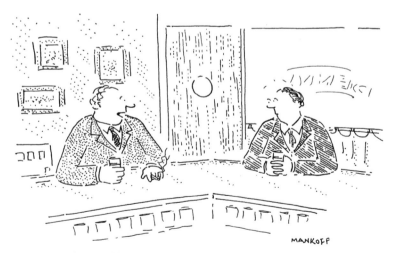

"See, the problem with doing things to prolong your life is that all the extra years come at the end, when you're old."

prepare good food. According to her husband, Karla's homemade sausages and cheesecake are famous in their village.

But now they eat mostly vegetable oil and high-fiber foods. When they buy a steak for a special occasion, they cut off all the fat.

"And that's the tasty part," Karla sighed. "If only the diet had lowered my cholesterol, but it didn't."

"Diet is not enough," the doctor said. "You also need pills."

Karla hated the diet, but it was nothing compared to the drug.

"You have to stand a little discomfort," the doctor told her.

The diet made it easy to slim down, and what was left of her appetite disappeared completely when she started the nauseating medication.

Add to this the demise of her positive attitude. She had looked forward to retirement with her husband, but now all seemed bleak. She felt she had nothing to look forward to.

Her cholesterol went down but not enough, the doctor said, and the dietician looked at her with great skepticism when Karla told her what she ate.

"It's impossible. You must have eaten more fat than that," the dietician scolded.

In fact, Karla had eaten some cheesecake the day before, but it hadn't been a pleasure; she felt terribly guilty afterwards.

Do you think that Karla is unique? Let me tell you about the result of a health project in Luleå, Sweden, headed by Birger Grahn, one of the general practitioners in the district. The aim of the study was to lower the incidence of coronary heart disease. Participants were sent a computerized letter containing a description of their "health profile." Afterwards Birgitta Olsson, a social scientist, questioned one hundred of the recipients.

Twenty-six of these healthy individuals said the letter frightened them. "It was like a shock," or "as if the world collapsed," some of them answered. One stated that she was "almost paralyzed."

Those with high cholesterol were the most frightened. "The risk that you will have a coronary in five years is estimated to be considerably higher than the average risk for inhabitants of Luleå of the same age and sex as you," the letter said.

When Birgitta Olsson asked again half a year later, after all the health-promoting activities had started, a further thirteen suffered from anxiety.[1]

You may think that anxiety about cholesterol is something peculiar to the Swedes, but that is not the case. According to a recent Gallup poll in the United States, 56 percent of all Americans worry about fat and cholesterol, 45 percent think that the food they like is not good for them, and 36 percent have guilt feelings when they eat the food they like.

Apart from the fact that worrying about your health may provoke heart trouble, all this stress and anxiety are unnecessary. Karla and millions of others around the world with high blood cholesterol do not know that the cholesterol campaign is medical quackery of the first order. In fact, the eminent American physician and scientist George Mann called the diet-heart idea "the greatest scientific deception of this century, perhaps of any century."

Unfortunately, Karla and millions of others do not know that high blood cholesterol is nothing to worry about.

This book has been written to give you and your doctor some facts about cholesterol and coronary heart disease (CHD). They are facts that even your doctor may not know because these facts have been misunderstood; or because many scientists, health authorities and representatives of the drug companies have suppressed them altogether.

To begin, let me tell you a little about how scientists work.

The scientific method

To bring a little order into a chaotic and hostile world, we try to find the laws that govern the "mess" that we observe. Medical researchers want to discover the threats against human life and health, and to know what causes disease and premature death, in order to cure or prevent these problems. To this end, we have developed a laborious but highly successful technique called the scientific method.

When we use the scientific method, the first step is to record all the facts about a disease. Who are the victims—men or women, young or old? How do they live and what do they do for a living? What do they eat and drink? What is the chemical makeup of their blood? How clean or dirty is the air they breathe? Scientists meticulously weigh, measure and analyze anything that may be of importance.

Every new piece of the puzzle leads us to speculate about the causes of the disease and to formulate a hypothesis—a theory that we must prove. To see if our hypothesis is correct, we test it in all possible ways. Is some factor present in all cases of the disease? Can the disease be produced by this factor, and can we prevent or cure the disease if we eliminate the factor?

If it doesn't pass all the tests, then our hypothesis is a bad one and must be rejected. Then we construct a new hypothesis that we hope will conform better to reality. We test and observe again. If necessary—and it often is necessary—we reformulate our hypothesis and repeat our tests a third and fourth and fifth time until, at last, we have a little nugget of pure truth in our hands. True scientists put the solution to a medical problem first and not the preservation of their own hypothesis, no matter how clever the hypothesis may seem or how proud of themselves they may be for creating it.

Scientists know that it is very rare for their first inspired thought to solve a scientific problem. Therefore, in our search for solutions, we scientists are as much interested in test results that destroy our hypothesis as we are in results that confirm it. And we do not blame anybody for a bad idea, providing that it is abandoned as soon as its flaws become obvious.

Defining our terms

This book is about the idea—the false idea—that a high level of cholesterol in the blood is the main cause of atherosclerosis and coronary heart disease. But what is atherosclerosis? And what is coronary heart disease?

When we grow old our arteries become stiff. The smooth muscle cells and the elastic fibers that surround our blood vessels when we are young are gradually replaced by more or less fibrous and rigid tissue. At the same time, or later on, cholesterol, various fats and even calcium become embedded in the blood vessel wall.

Arteries probably become stiff as a protective measure, to prevent the pressure of the blood inside them from causing them to widen too much.[2,3] Thus, the remodeling of the arteries does not occur evenly. It is most pronounced where the strain to the artery wall is highest, for instance, where the blood vessels branch. Such localized thickening is called an atheroma or plaque. Atherosclerosis increases with age, as does the blood pressure, and atherosclerosis is most pronounced in individuals with high blood pressure.

The fact that arteries that are prevented from widening, such as those that pass through the bony channels in the skull and the few branches that pass through the heart muscle (most branches lie on the surface of the heart), never become sclerotic also suggests that stiffening of the arteries may be a protective measure. Furthermore, veins never become sclerotic, probably because the blood pressure in veins is very low. If a surgeon replaces a clogged artery with a section of vein, however, this vein, now exposed to the high arterial blood pressure, soon becomes sclerotic.

For unknown reasons, in some people the embedding of cholesterol in the arterial wall becomes irregular and protrudes into the interior of the artery. Sometimes these localized protrusions, called raised lesions, even change into a material similar to limestone. The embedding of cholesterol and lime may also progress until the vessel becomes so narrow that the heart gets too little blood and thus too little oxygen. It is these constrictions that are considered to be the cause of heart attacks, either directly, or by starting the formation of a clot.

When the blood flow to the heart becomes insufficient, symptoms of discomfort radiating from the chest may result, especially if the heart's need for oxygen is increased during exercise. These symptoms are called angina; they disappear if you stop exercising. But if the blood flow is totally arrested, or if it is reduced too much for too a long time, the part of the heart that is supplied by the obstructed branch of the artery will die. This is called a heart attack, or a coronary, or, more precisely, a myocardial infarction. Angina and myocardial infarction taken together is what we call coronary heart disease, often shortened to CHD.

Atherosclerosis is said to be the cause of coronary heart disease, but the matter is not that simple. Anything that obstructs the coronary arteries may produce coronary heart disease. Studies of the hearts of people who have died from a heart attack have revealed that in about a fifth of the patients there is no evidence of coronary atherosclerosis. The arrested blood flow in such cases may have been due to a spasm of the artery, or to a clot that dissolved before death, but we don't know for sure.

To further complicate the story, a coronary artery may be totally obstructed without any symptoms and without any damage to the heart. The explanation is that the fine branches of the three coronary arteries communicate with each other. If blockage of an artery develops slowly enough, the communicating branches gradually widen, allowing the neighbor to carry more of the blood supply.[4]

Thus, a myocardial infarction may occur even though the coronary arteries are totally normal, and coronary heart disease may be absent even though the coronary arteries may be completely blocked. Obviously, atherosclerosis and coronary heart disease are separate conditions, but many researchers have confused our thinking by considering them as one.

The Diet-Heart idea

In the search for the causes of atherosclerosis and heart disease, researchers since the early 1950s have focused on a single hypothesis or idea. This is the diet-heart idea, sometimes called the lipid hypothesis. As I will explain in this book, the diet-heart idea is a hypothesis that has not passed the basic scientific tests, a hypothesis that is filled with obvious absurdities.

The diet-heart idea is not scientifically sound, but it survives. In fact, the diet-heart idea is hopelessly incorrect, but it seems to have eternal life. It lives on because the researchers who created it and defend it—I will call them the proponents—have not followed the principles dictated by the scientific method.

Those principles demand open-mindedness and objectivity, but the proponents of the diet-heart hypothesis routinely belittle, deny or explain away any scientific observations that contradict their idea. They take the weakest association that supports their idea and call it strong evidence, and they refuse to consider any conflicting observation. In the process, logic becomes as remote as a town in Siberia. Proponents of the diet-heart idea often ask, "What is wrong?" but when they ask this, they mean what is wrong with the conflicting evidence and not with their pet hypothesis. Masses of valid scientific evidence should have destroyed the diet-heart idea by now. Yet, like the ancient Greek Hydra, a mythological monster that grew new heads whenever its old ones were chopped off, the cholesterol Hydra continues its life as if nothing had happened.

But before we look at evidence that should destroy the diet-heart idea, let's first consider what that idea is.

According to diet-heart proponents, coronary heart disease is the third and final step of a three-step process. In the first step, or so the proponents claim, the amount and the type of fat in our diet determines the level of cholesterol in our blood. They say that if we eat an atherogenic diet, our blood cholesterol will be high. And by an atherogenic diet they mean a diet containing

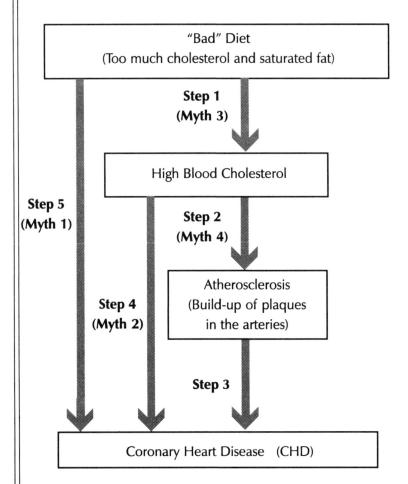

THE DIET-HEART IDEA

"Bad" Diet
(Too much cholesterol and saturated fat)

**Step 1
(Myth 3)**

High Blood Cholesterol

**Step 5
(Myth 1)**

**Step 2
(Myth 4)**

Atherosclerosis
(Build-up of plaques
in the arteries)

**Step 4
(Myth 2)**

Step 3

Coronary Heart Disease   (CHD)

The Diet-Heart Idea: The short arrows (1, 2 and 3) represent the three steps of the hypothesis. The long arrows (4 and 5) stand for logical (or seemingly logical) consequences of the short arrows.

too much cholesterol and saturated fat (found mainly in animal products, such as meat, milk, eggs but also in palm oil and coconut oil) and too little polyunsaturated fat (found mainly in marine animals and commercial vegetable oils). According to the proponents, step two occurs because high blood cholesterol is the main cause of atherosclerosis. And in step three, or so the proponents claim, atherosclerosis causes coronary heart disease by blocking the blood vessels of the heart. The idea sounds simple, and most of us are familiar with it after reading about low-fat recipes and low-fat diets for years in popular magazines and newspapers.

At first glance, the diet-heart hypothesis does indeed appear simple, logical and well-founded. It is also an attractive idea, because it almost promises that death from coronary heart disease can be prevented. If animal fat and high blood cholesterol are the villains, then cholesterol-lowering diets and cholesterol-lowering medicines appear to be wise choices. It's easy to understand why doctors, politicians, pharmaceutical companies and the manufacturers of vegetable oils and low-fat frozen dinners have embraced the diet-heart idea.

But very few people know that it is built on nothing more than circumstantial evidence. Nobody has ever seen the villains in action. There are many diseases that we have explained from circumstantial evidence but only when all the evidence has pointed in the same direction. As for the diet-heart hypothesis, the evidence is contradictory and confusing. In fact, huge numbers of published medical studies reveal results that are totally at odds with this idea.

For many years, millions of people have endured a tasteless, tedious diet or have suffered serious side effects from cholesterol-lowering drugs because of the diet-heart idea. And billions of dollars have been spent in vain because previous research, reviewed in the chapters to come, had already demonstrated the diet-heart hypothesis to be completely worthless.

Medical experts and health authorities will criticize this book and its author because their prestige is at stake. They will probably describe the author as unscientific or incompetent, and they will say that prestigious committees all over the world have decided that the diet-heart idea has been proved beyond all reasonable doubt.

This book is written for people who can think for themselves. And if you find that something I have written seems too incredible, please consult the references. Then go to a university library and read the original papers yourself. By doing this systematically, as I have done, you will not only see that I am correct, but you will also learn more about cholesterol and the heart than most researchers have. Judging from their papers, many of those researchers seem to have read only reviews, and reviews written by the proponents are notoriously unreliable. In the chapters to follow, I shall give you many examples of misquotations from such reviews.

One of my objections to the diet-heart idea is that its proponents are selective about their data. They lean on studies that support their idea—or that they claim, not always truthfully, support it—and ignore those that contradict them.

One of the proponents once accused me of pointing only to studies that do not support the diet-heart idea and, thus, of using a technique similar to the one the proponents use.

He was right.

What he failed to remember is that, if a scientific hypothesis is sound, it must agree with *all* observations. A hypothesis is not like a sports event, where the team with the greatest number of points wins the game. Even *one* observation that does not support a hypothesis is enough to disprove it. The proponents of a scientific idea have the burden of proof on *their* shoulders. The opponent does not have to present an alternative idea; his task is only to find the weakness in the hypothesis. If there is only one proof against it, one proof that cannot be denied and that is based on reliable scientific observations, the hypothesis must be rejected. And the diet-heart idea is filled with features that have repeatedly been proven false.

The history of science is one in which many attractive ideas have been discarded when found to conflict with observed fact. For instance, the earth was considered to be a flat planet around which the sun and the other planets revolved. Anyone could ascertain this by looking at the horizontal skyline. And, with his own eyes, anyone could see how the sun, like the moon, circled around the earth.

Our ancestors did not know better because they had only the naked eye and lacked the technology needed to discover the truth. But the proponents of the diet-heart idea ought to know. Instead, their cocksure writings demonstrate that for them the idea has become a fact, the cholesterol earth is flat.

Or is it only a game? Those of you who read this book will realize that scientists who support the diet-heart idea and who are honest must be ignorant, either because they have failed to understand what they have read or else, by blindly following the authorities, they have failed to check the accuracy of the studies written by those authorities. But some scientists must surely have realized that the diet-heart idea is impossible and yet, for various reasons, have chosen to keep the idea alive.

In both politics and religion, ideas can be more powerful than any army. In medicine, ideas can also have powerful consequences.

Let us now explore a medical hypothesis, the diet-heart idea, which, although it seriously conflicts with the laws of logic, has dominated scientific thinking for many years—with many unfortunate consequences.

Myth 1

High-Fat Foods Cause Heart Disease

Some circumstantial evidence is very strong, as when you find a trout in the milk.

Henry David Thoreau (1817-1862)

A challenge

In 1953 Ancel Keys, director of the Laboratory of Physiological Hygiene at the University of Minnesota, published a paper that served as an early kickoff for the cholesterol campaign.[1]

The US Public Health Service's outlook is too limited, he wrote; any major disease should be prevented, not just those of infectious or occupational origin.

It doesn't matter that the necessary measures are not yet known, he argued. The mere hope that the incidence of a disease may be altered is sufficient reason to invest money and manpower in its prevention.

What Dr. Keys had in mind was coronary heart disease. This disease is a threat, he continued. While all other diseases are decreasing in the United States, there has been a steady upward trend in the death rate from coronary heart disease. On this particular point, the Americans are inferior to other countries; in the US, for example, four to five times more die from a heart attack than in Italy.

While Dr. Keys may have had initial reservations about which measures could prevent heart disease, he quickly put them aside;

he already knew what to do. He considered a defeatist attitude about coronary heart disease to be despicable. According to Dr. Keys, it was "abundantly clear" that heart attacks could be prevented. And he already knew what the preventive measures should be. If the Italians could do it, so could Americans, he added. "These figures are a challenge."

Remember that Dr. Keys was directing these words to Americans, a proud people for whom the word "aggressive" is a word of honor, in health care as in other matters. In the US, more diagnostic tests are performed than in any other country; surgery is preferred over drugs and, when drugs are chosen, high doses and strong preparations are used.[2] Ancel Keys' words did not go unheeded.

According to Dr. Keys, high-fat food was the culprit. His proof was a diagram, published in 1953, which showed a close correlation between the total intake of fat and the death rates from coronary heart disease in six countries. (See Figure 1A.) The points of the diagram lay almost perfectly on the upward curve of CHD deaths, so perfectly that the curve he drew looked more like the result of an experiment in physics than biology. If you extend the curve to the left it intersects the origin (the intersection of the x- and y-axes), thus suggesting that if you completely avoid high-fat food, you will never have a heart attack.

One year later *The Lancet*, one of the world's most prestigious medical journals, published the following statement: "The curve shows an almost convincing relationship between the fat content of the food and the risk of dying from coronary heart disease."

But why did Dr. Keys limit his data to a mere six countries? At that time information was available from 22 countries. The reason is that if all of the countries were included, the association became rather weak. The death rate from coronary heart disease in Finland, for instance, was seven times that of Mexico, although fat consumption in the two nations was almost the same. (See Figure 1B.)

Are consumption data accurate?

Let us have another look at the graphs in Figures 1A and 1B. They are similar to graphs presented again and again by proponents of the diet-heart idea. What do the figures really mean?

First, "Calories from Fat" does not mean the amount of fat eaten in each country, only the amount available for consumption. The data used in Figures 1A and 1B represent the sum of the fat produced in the country plus the amount imported minus food used for purposes other than human nutrition. This may not give an accurate picture, however, because it does not take into account the amount of fat that is never delivered to the consumers, that is lost, stolen, eaten by rats or mice or spoiled because of bad storage. Furthermore, some of it is eaten by dogs, cats and other pet animals; some is thrown away in the kitchen or left on the plate. In the US, where eating fat is considered almost a sin, a great deal of fat certainly disappears that way. In poor countries, however, where famine is a greater threat than overweight or heart disease, it is not so. Here, the diet even includes brain and bone marrow, both of which are crammed with animal fat and cholesterol.

Thus, the figures for fat consumption in various countries are unreliable, to put it mildly. But the figures for heart mortality, those on the vertical axis in Figures 1A and 1B, are even more erroneous.

Are death certificates true?

When statisticians write their reports about numbers and causes of death in a population, they consult the death certificates. Do you think that what is written on this piece of paper is the truth and nothing but the truth?

Certainly not. Again and again great differences have been found between the diagnosis set by the doctor while the patient was alive and the findings at autopsy. Even doctors with access to modern diagnostic equipment put the wrong diagnosis on the

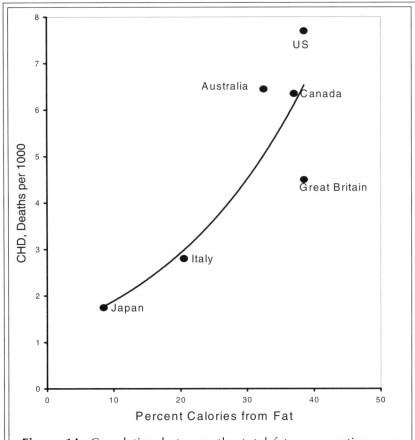

Figure 1A. Correlation between the total fat consumption as a percent of total calorie consumption, and mortality from coronary heart disease in six countries. Data from Keys.[1]

death certificate in one out of three cases.[4] For instance, most doctors consider sudden, unexpected death to be caused by a heart attack due to coronary heart disease. Dr. George Lundberg from the University of California and Professor Gerhard Voigt from the University of Lund, Sweden, showed this to be wrong. In 51 percent of such cases, the cause of death was something else.[5]

The situation is no better when patients have actually died of heart attacks. Drs. Edwin Zarling, Harold Sexton and Pervis Milnor from Memphis, Tennessee, found that among 100 pa-

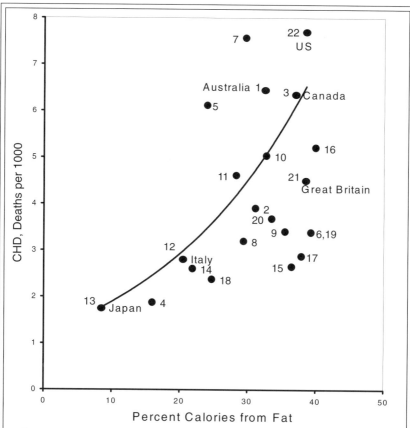

Figure 1B. Same as Figure 1A, but including all countries where data were available when Dr. Keys published his paper. 1. Australia 2. Austria 3. Canada 4. Ceylon 5. Chile 6. Denmark 7. Finland 8. France 9. West Germany 10. Ireland. 11. Israel 12. Italy 13. Japan 14. Mexico 15. Holland 16. New Zealand 17. Norway 18. Portugal 19. Sweden 20. Switzerland 21. Great Britain 22. USA.   Data from Yerushalmy and Hilleboe.[3]

tients who died from a heart attack according to the postmortem, only 53 had a correct diagnosis before they died.[6]

These studies were not performed in small local hospitals but at university hospitals where experienced academic doctors had access to the finest diagnostic tools that modern medical science can provide.

Maybe you think that it is unimportant what the doctor diagnoses as cause of death because mistakes will be corrected by the coroner. But postmortems are performed in only a minority of cases; in the US in one out of five cases, in other countries much less often.

So, if the diagnostic accuracy is that bad in a modern, western hospital, how do you think it is in poor countries where the cause of death is rarely written down by doctors, much less by a coroner?

But even frequent postmortems are no guarantee of a correct diagnosis. This was amply demonstrated by the British professors Reid and Rose.[7] They collected summaries from the hospital records of ten patients who had died from various heart, kidney and lung diseases. Except for the diagnoses, the summaries contained all information relevant to the causes of the patients' deaths, including results of physical and laboratory examinations, statements from the X-ray department and the postmortem descriptions. Then, a number of experienced, academically trained doctors from university hospitals in Norway, England and the US were told: "Read the records and write the death certificates!"

Any scientist who considers statistics based on death certificates as a source of truth should look carefully at the study by Drs. Reid and Rose. Coronary heart disease was used as a diagnosis by the American doctors 33 percent more often than by the English doctors, and 50 percent more often than by the Norwegian doctors.

Someone who is not a physician may find it odd that doctors from countries with similar medical traditions and education systems act so differently when they put a diagnosis on the death certificate. The explanation is that there may be serious changes in many organs in a dying person, but on the death certificate and in the statistical tables there is room for only one diagnosis. Thus, in complicated cases American doctors, for unknown reasons, are inclined to blame death on changes in the vessels to the heart, whereas English and Norwegian doctors may instead hold lung or brain diseases responsible. Interestingly, the official death statistics from these three countries reflect these tendencies.[8]

If death is labeled so differently in the US, England and Norway where the medical education is similar, how is it labeled in countries such as Japan, Sri Lanka or Mexico where the culture and medical traditions are fundamentally dissimilar?

Clearly, official death statistics are based on diagnoses that, in at least half of the cases, are plain wrong, and if they are not wrong, they do not tell the whole truth.

Television—a risk factor?

But let us assume that heart attacks are more common in countries where people eat large amounts of fat. What does that mean?

From Table 1A, you can see that factors other than consumption of fat are associated with heart disease. The correlation coefficient in the right-hand column of the table tells how well various factors are related to the number of deaths from heart attacks in the countries that were studied. The largest coefficient is 1, the weakest is zero. The table thus tells us that in countries where heart attacks are common (meaning where the diagnosis of coronary heart disease is commonly used) people eat more protein, fat, cholesterol and sugar. They also smoke more cigarettes and buy more cars than in countries where heart attacks are less common.

What the statistics actually tell you is that the risk of having the diagnosis of coronary heart disease written on one's death certificate is greater for people in prosperous countries than for people in poor countries. Therefore, anything that follows with or from prosperity is automatically associated with mortality from coronary heart disease. Calories from animal fat, for instance, are more expensive than calories from other nutrients; more animal fat is therefore available for consumption in prosperous countries than in poor countries. And since the cause of death is called coronary heart disease more often in prosperous countries than in poor ones, the intake of animal fat becomes statistically associated with the number of deaths from heart disease.

Thus, population studies may point to factors that are *associated with* a certain diagnosis on death certificates but they cannot tell us the cause of the disease; only experiments can. Factors that are statistically associated with a disease are called *risk factors.* A risk factor *may* be the cause of the disease, but most often it is not. Several hundred risk factors are known for coronary heart disease, including smoking, overweight, high blood pressure, lack of exercise, psychological stress, baldness, snoring and eating too much or too little of a steadily increasing number of various food items, but the cause of the disease is still unknown. Table 1A lists only a few examples of risk factors for coronary heart disease.

Table 1A. Correlation coefficients between various consumption factors and mortality in coronary heart disease for men age 55-64 in 22 countries.

Factor	Correlation Coefficient
Number of cigarettes sold per inhabitant	0.64
Number of cars sold per 100 inhabitants	0.58
Total consumption of protein*	0.72
Consumption of animal protein*	0.73
Total consumption of fat*	0.56
Consumption of animal fat*	0.65
Consumption of cholesterol*	0.69
Consumption of sugar*	0.68

*Amount available for consumption
Data from Yerushalmy and Hilleboe.[3]

Because a risk factor and the cause of a disease may stem from a common factor, such as a country's prosperity, it is self-evident that the elimination of the risk factor does not automatically prevent the disease; the main cause is still there.

Let us assume that the real cause of coronary heart disease is car exhaust. (This is most likely totally wrong but that doesn't matter; I have made this assumption only to demonstrate how factors that vary together may create false associations). More people are exposed to car exhaust in prosperous countries because cars are more common in prosperous countries and, as we assumed that coronary heart disease was due to car exhaust, heart attacks should also be more common. Logically, death rates from coronary disease in various countries become associated with the number of cars sold. But people in prosperous countries buy many other things more often than people in poor countries, such as television sets, and thus the coronary death rates also become associated with the number of television sets sold. You may therefore call "possession of a television set" a risk factor although it is obvious that television sets do not cause heart disease. (See Figure 1C.) Clearly, it is a bad idea to throw the television set out the window to save the heart.

To carry our example one step further, see Figure 1D, which shows the correlation between the tax rate and death from heart disease in the municipal tax districts of the county of Stockholm, Sweden. The graph implies that if the municipal tax rate is lowered to 9.55 percent, no one will die from a heart attack—a challenge to all politicians!

People with yellow fingers die from heart attacks more often than others. "Yellow fingers" is therefore a risk factor for coronary heart disease. But it doesn't help to scrub away the yellow color, because the discoloration is due to cigarette smoking. The cause of coronary heart disease is not the yellow color, but either the smoke from the tobacco or the paper, or the mental stress that starts the habit of smoking, or a factor associated with the habit of smoking or the feeling generated by nicotine.

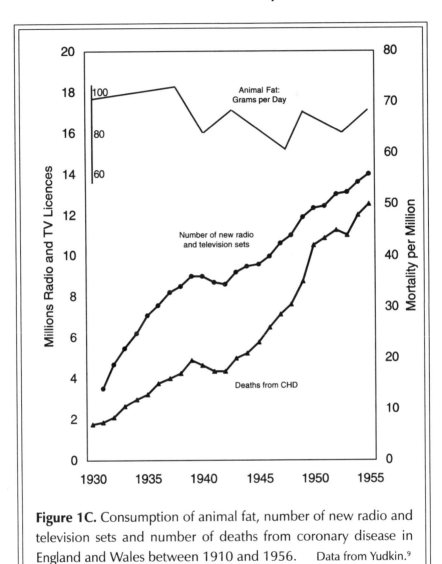

Figure 1C. Consumption of animal fat, number of new radio and television sets and number of deaths from coronary disease in England and Wales between 1910 and 1956.　Data from Yudkin.[9]

One of the biggest problems with the diet-heart idea is that proponents fail to distinguish between *risk factors* (like animal fat, television sets and yellow fingers) and *cause*. Risk factors do not necessarily produce disease. But most diet-heart supporters rarely explain this distinction. Instead, they consider every new risk factor as something that should be reduced or eliminated.

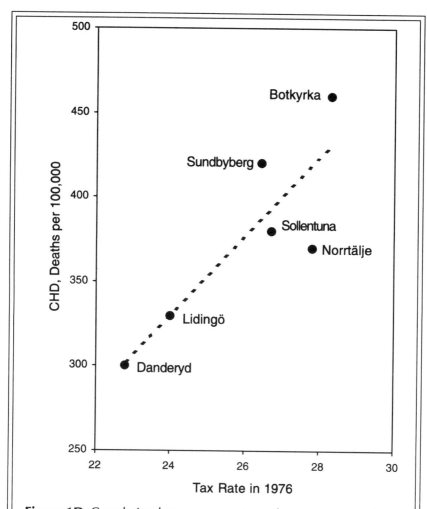

Figure 1D. Correlation between tax rate and coronary mortality in the municipal tax districts of the county of Stockholm, Sweden. A logical conclusion from this figure is that if the municipal tax rate is lowered to 9.55 percent, no one will die from a heart attack—a challenge to all politicians!

Seven random countries

To prove his idea about dietary fat, Dr. Keys organized a study of coronary heart disease in seven countries.[10] To this end he selected sixteen local populations in the Netherlands, Yugoslavia, Finland, Japan, Greece, Italy and the US. In cooperation with local doctors, scientists and health authorities, researchers investigated anything that might conceivably cause coronary heart disease. They followed men between the age of 40 and 59 for about five years, and recorded all heart symptoms and all deaths.

In each country investigators studied two or three groups of people. Researchers looked at diet, measured blood pressure and weighed all participants. Participants were also asked how much they smoked and exercised.

The conclusion from this gigantic project was that the factor most likely to predict the number of heart attacks in a country was the amount of animal fat people ate in that country. (In striking contrast to Keys' previous study, no association was found with the total fat consumption!) In countries where people ate lots of animal fat, heart attacks were common; in countries where people ate small amounts of animal fat, heart attacks were rare.

But *within* the countries the number of heart attacks showed no correlation with the diet. Let's consider two Finnish populations, one from North Karelia and one from Turku.

At the beginning of the study, 42 out of 817 men from North Karelia had coronary heart disease while in the district of Turku only 15 of 860 had CHD. During the next five years, 16 men died from a heart attack in North Karelia, but only four in the district of Turku. Taking all factors into consideration, heart attacks occurred five times more often in North Karelia than in the district of Turku.

If you think that the natives lived especially carelessly in North Karelia, you are wrong. The living conditions in the two areas were practically identical. In both districts, people lived isolated lives as farmers or lumberjacks, their body weight and height were identical as were their blood cholesterol levels,[11] they smoked equally as much and they ate the same amount of polyunsaturated fat. Blood pressure levels were slightly higher in

North Karelia, and the inhabitants also ate slightly more animal fat than those living in Turku.

Dr. Keys declared that coronary heart disease was five times more common in Finland than in Japan because of large differences in the food, but he did not explain why coronary heart disease was five times more common in eastern than in western Finland even though the difference between the common risk factors was only marginal. He mentioned this disconcerting fact as a minor, abnormal finding, which he believed (erroneously) would be explained by further studies.

This double standard is common among the proponents of the diet-heart idea. Observations that support the theory are trumpeted as positive proofs while unsupportive findings, if they are mentioned at all, are considered as "rare exceptions" or "something which cannot yet be explained."

Ups and downs in statistics

To determine whether the fat in our food has any influence on our proneness to heart attacks, it is instructive to study how the eating habits in a country have changed during a period of time and to ask whether the number of heart attacks has changed in the expected direction. If animal fat is an important cause of coronary heart disease, then the number of heart attacks should increase during periods when consumption of animal fat is also increasing; and it should decrease when less animal fat is eaten.

But even if these figures follow each other up and down, we have not proved that eating animal fat is the cause of the increasing mortality. Again, an unknown factor could create parallel changes in fat intake and heart mortality. Let me give an example.

During World War II people in Finland, Norway, Sweden and Great Britain died less often from heart attacks than before the war. According to Haquin Malmroos, a professor of medicine in Lund, Sweden, this is because people ate less animal fat.

But other things of importance to the problem of heart dis-

KNOW YOUR FATS

The fats and oils in our food, and the fats in our bodies, are composed of fatty acids—chains of carbon atoms with hydrogen filling the unused carbon bonds.

A fatty acid is *saturated* when all available carbon bonds are occupied by a hydrogen atom. Saturated fats are highly stable because all the carbon-atom linkages are filled—or saturated—with hydrogen. This means that they do not normally go rancid, even when heated for cooking purposes. They are straight in form and hence pack together easily, so that they form a solid or semi-solid fat at room temperature. Your body makes saturated fatty acids from carbohydrates and uses them in a number of ways. Dietary saturated fats are also supplied by animal fats such as butter, lard and tallow, and by tropical oils such as coconut oil.

Monounsaturated fatty acids have one double bond in the form of two carbon atoms double-bonded to each other and, there-fore, lack two hydrogen atoms. Your body makes monounsat-urated fatty acids from saturated fatty acids and uses them in a number of ways. Monounsaturated fats have a kink or bend at the position of the double bond so that they do not pack together as easily as saturated fats. Thus, they tend to be liquid at room temperature. Like saturated fats, they are relatively stable. They do not go rancid easily and can be used in cooking. The monoun-saturated fatty acid most commonly found in our food is oleic acid, the main component of olive oil as well as the oils from almonds, pecans, cashews, peanuts, palm fruit and avocados.

Polyunsaturated fatty acids have two or more pairs of double bonds and, therefore, lack four or more hydrogen atoms. The two polyunsaturated fatty acids found most frequently in our foods are double unsaturated linoleic acid, with two double bonds—also called omega-6; and triple unsaturated linolenic acid, with three double bonds—also called omega-3. (The omega number indicates the position of the first double bond.) Your body cannot make these fatty acids, which is why they are called "essential." We must obtain our essential fatty acids or EFAs from the foods we eat. The polyunsaturated fatty acids have kinks or turns at the position of the double bond and, hence, do not pack together easily. They are liquid, even when refrigerated. The unpaired electrons at the double bonds makes these oils highly reactive. They go rancid easily, particularly omega-3 linolenic acid, and must be treated with care.

Polyunsaturated fatty acids are found in almost all whole foods including fish, meat, eggs, dairy products, fruit, vegetables, grains and legumes. Before the advent of modern vegetable oils, mankind consumed small amounts of fresh, undamaged polyunsaturated fatty acids found naturally as a component of his food. Consumption of polyunsaturated fatty acids is much higher today because vegetable oils are used widely as cooking oils and in salad dressings, baked goods and snack foods.

Polyunsaturated oils should never be heated—yet during the extraction process these oils are subjected to very high temperatures that encourage rancidity and the formation of many harmful breakdown products. Commercial vegetable oils are also deodorized to remove the smell of rancidity.

Enig MG. *Know Your Fats: The Complete Primer for Understanding the Nutrition of Fats, Oils, and Cholesterol.* Bethesda Press, Bethesda, MD, 2000.

ease occurred during the war. For instance, people's body weight and blood pressure went down considerably, fewer people smoked, and the lack of gasoline for cars and other machinery may have favored a healthier way of life. A common denominator of the war was lack of goods—including a lack of rich food, for instance—but also lack of other nutrients and of gasoline and of cigarettes.

Nobody knows which of these factors, if any, caused the decrease in heart disease. The explanation that people ate less

animal fat is unlikely because it has never been possible to lower
the death rate from coronary heart disease with a low-fat diet in
experiments of the same length as World War II.

Furthermore, the mortality curves turned upwards again
long before the increase in animal fat consumption took place.

Thus, although a risk factor changes in parallel to the death
rate, that still does not mean that the risk factor is necessarily
the cause. But if the risk factor *is* the cause, its rise and fall must
be reflected, with *no* exceptions, in the rise and fall in the death
rate from the disease. If heart attacks are caused by eating too
much animal fat, heart attacks should, of course, become more
frequent when people start to eat more of such fat. Likewise, if
people change their diet and eat less animal fat, fewer heart attacks should occur. But this is not what happened.

From World War I up to the 1980s, the number of deaths
from heart attacks increased substantially in most countries while
the intake of animal fat decreased or was unchanged. For instance, the death rate from cardiovascular diseases in middle-
aged Yugoslavians increased three to four times between 1955
and 1965, while the intake of fat decreased by 25 percent.[12]

In England the intake of animal fat has been relatively stable
since at least 1910 while the number of heart attacks increased
ten times between 1930 and 1970.[9]

In the US, coronary mortality increased about ten times between 1930 and 1960, leveled off during the '60s and has since
decreased slowly. During the decline of heart mortality the consumption of animal fat declined also, but during the thirty years
of sharply rising coronary mortality the consumption of animal
fat decreased.[13]

In the town of Framingham, Massachusetts, the number of
fatal heart attacks went down during the decline of animal fat
consumption, but the number of nonfatal heart attacks increased
during the same period.[14] The authors of the Framingham report explained this discrepancy by saying that it takes much
longer to lower the number of nonfatal heart attacks than to lower

the number of fatal cases.[15] (A much better explanation is that more people survive a heart attack today because of improved treatment.)

In Japan the number of fatal heart attacks between 1950 and 1970 increased, as did the intake of animal fat, an apparent confirmation of the diet-heart idea. But the increase in coronary mortality was seen only in those above the age of 70 and especially above 80. In the latter age group, the increase in coronary mortality more than counterbalanced the decrease in the other age groups. In other words, younger Japanese people died less often of coronary disease, although they ate more animal fat. During the same period mortality from most diseases decreased in Japan. Thus, the increasing death rate from coronary disease among old people in Japan could not be caused by an increased intake of animal fat; if it were, the number of coronary deaths should have increased in all age groups. The explanation is that the general health in Japan has improved steadily since the war, as has the mean length of life. Many more have become old, and since coronary heart disease is a disease of old age, the death rate due to heart disease has, of course, increased.[16]

This torpedo against the diet-heart idea was presented as the first paper at an international conference in 1981. Yet the paper caused no backlash in the scientific community. Instead, Dr. Kimura, the author of the paper, concluded: ". . . if this food supply and nutrient intake pattern continues the same evolution in Japan, incidence of ischemic heart disease will increase in the future." The conference then continued with paper after paper acknowledging the diet-heart idea.[16b]

Contrary to Dr. Kimura's prophecy, since 1970 the number of fatal heart attacks has continued to decline in Japan in all age groups, in spite of a continuing increase in animal fat consumption.[16c,17]

While the death rate from coronary disease increased in most countries after World War II, it decreased in Switzerland. If this decrease had been preceded by a decline in the intake of animal fat, Switzerland would have been a model for health care in other countries. But the diet-heart proponents never mention Switzerland because during the decline in heart mortality, the Swiss intake of animal fat increased by 20 percent.[18]

The shepherds of Kenya

The many exceptions to Ancel Keys' hypothesis indicate that something in the Western lifestyle other than consumption of animal fat is the cause of coronary heart disease. To be absolutely sure, it is necessary to study people who eat just as much animal fat as we do but who are not exposed to the menaces of Western civilization. If diet were the most important factor, people in such countries would have equally high cholesterol and would die just as often from heart attacks as we do.

In the early 1960s, Professor George Mann and his team from Vanderbilt University in Nashville took a mobile laboratory to Kenya in Africa in order to study the Masai people.[19] At that time, the diet-heart idea was gaining triumphant success throughout the scientific world. Professor Mann had heard that the Masai people ate nothing but milk, blood and meat. Wouldn't it be a good idea to test the diet-heart idea on the Kenyan plateau? Shortly before and with the same purpose, Dr. Gerald Shaper from the Makerere University of Uganda had traveled a little farther north to study another tribe, the Samburus.[20]

The Samburus and the Masai are slender people who have survived as shepherds for thousands of years. Their life is free from the mental stress and competition of Western civilization, but you cannot call it comfortable. Every day they walk or run many miles with their cattle, searching for food and water.

Their own diet is extreme. According to their view, vegetables and fiber are food for cows; they themselves consume only milk, meat and blood, or at least the younger men do. A male Samburu may drink over one gallon of milk each day, which works out to well over one pound of butterfat. He has never heard about the cholesterol campaign and, therefore, he drinks the creamy milk as it is, without removing the fat, which means that his intake of animal fat is far above that of most Western people. His intake of cholesterol is also high, especially during periods when he adds two to four pounds of meat to his daily diet of milk.[20]

The Masai drink "only" half a gallon of milk each day. However, they eat more meat than the Samburus. Their parties are sheer orgies of meat; on such occasions four to ten pounds of meat per person is not unusual, according to Professor Mann.

If the diet-heart idea were correct, coronary heart disease would be epidemic in Kenya. But Professor Mann found that the Masai do not die from heart disease—although they might die from laughter if they heard about the campaign against foods containing cholesterol and saturated fat.

But this was not the only surprise. The cholesterol of the Masai tribesmen was not sky-high as Mann had expected; it was very low. In fact, their cholesterol was among the lowest ever measured in the world, about 50 percent lower than the value of most Americans.

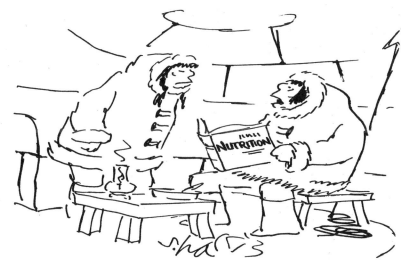

It appears that our diet is almost 100 percent cholesterol.
That appears to be very, very, very bad.

Another cholesterol safari

Now to Dr. Bruce Taylor from Chicago. He was the first scientist to induce a heart attack in an ape by cholesterol feeding. (See Chapter 5.) The papers about the Samburu and the Masai tribesmen were published shortly after Dr. Taylor's successful experiment. Certainly he must have asked himself why the cholesterol of his laboratory animals skyrocketed on their high-fat diet, but not the cholesterol of the Masai and the Samburu. To answer this question he set out for Kenya with his own expedition a few years later.

Like other mammals, our bodies produce cholesterol day and night. When we eat lots of cholesterol or animal fat, our own production of cholesterol decreases automatically. If we eat only a little, our production increases. This mechanism keeps the cholesterol level in the blood fairly constant and is the reason it is so difficult to lower cholesterol with diet.

After his investigations, Dr. Taylor reached an unusual conclusion about this balancing mechanism in the Masai. According to Dr. Taylor, the African tribes do not contradict the diet-heart idea because their ability to reduce their own cholesterol production is superior to that of other people. Because the Masai have been isolated from other tribes for many thousands of years, they have developed this ability so well that it has been built into their genes, Dr. Taylor said. Dr. Taylor and his colleagues considered their results so important that they published them, with minor variations, in four different scientific journals.[21]

In science there are often alternative explanations to a new observation, and most scientists therefore discuss which model or hypothesis best fits the new piece of evidence. But Dr. Taylor did not. He could have considered the possibility that it is not the Masai who are superior to others in reducing their cholesterol production but, instead, we who are inferior, perhaps because of environmental factors, perhaps because we are less active than the Masai or perhaps because of something we haven't yet imagined. But he did not.

It would have been possible to get an answer to these questions if he had continued his expedition to the city of Nairobi and studied the Masai there to see whether some factor associated with the more comfortable lifestyle of a big city might have increased their cholesterol. This method is often used by the defenders of the diet-heart idea to demonstrate that low cholesterol goes up when people from poor, undeveloped countries, where fat consumption is presumed to be low, move to a more prosperous and technologically developed country, where fat consumption is presumed to be high.[22]

But in this case, the study concerned human beings who already ate record-breaking amounts of animal fat. After migration to Nairobi their diet most probably became more diversified and, if the diet-heart idea were true, their blood cholesterol should have become even lower.

What had happened to the cholesterol of the urbanized Masai people? Why didn't Dr. Taylor and his colleagues proceed to Nairobi to get an answer to this simple question? Dr. Taylor's explanation that the low cholesterol of the Masai is due to genetics is not valid. Acquired properties are not transferred to people's descendants. This idea was abandoned as scientifically wrong many years ago. An inborn metabolic trait—in this case the ability to reduce the body's own production of cholesterol when there are large amounts of cholesterol in the diet—is either present in the genes, or it arises by mutation. If the property is important for survival, the number of individuals with this property increases over time and eventually these people may outnumber those without it. But this will happen only if the inborn trait improves survival before sexual maturity. Individuals with a trait that protects them against a disease that strikes after sexual maturity, such as coronary heart disease, do not outnumber individuals without this trait because the latter transfer their defective genes to their children before they develop the disease.

And, contrary to Dr. Taylor's statements, the Masai are not an isolated tribe. They are warlike people who have taken cattle and women from neighboring tribes for thousands of years. In this way they have achieved a steady genetic renewal in their cattle and in themselves.

But what finally proved that Dr. Taylor was wrong was a study performed by Dr. José Day at St. Mary's Hospital in London of Masai living in the big city of Nairobi. Again, if the low cholesterol of the Masai were inherited, it should have been even lower in Nairobi, because here their diet would most likely include lower amounts of animal fat than the diet of the Masai tribesmen. But the mean cholesterol level in 26 males in Nairobi was 25 percent higher than that of their cattle-breeding kinsmen in the countryside![23]

Dr. Taylor's genetic explanation has been popular among proponents of the diet-heart idea, such as Dr. Keys. He wrote: ". . . the fact is that the peculiarities of those primitive nomads have no relevance to diet-cholesterol-coronary heart disease relationships in other populations,"[24] but he did not explain why they "have no relevance."

Dr. Taylor studied not only blood cholesterol but also atherosclerosis in the Masai. It was important to show that their low cholesterol level protected the Masai from atherosclerosis. Ten aortas from deceased Masais were sent to New York where the pathologists said that atherosclerosis was almost absent.

But Professor Mann studied a much greater number of hearts and aortas from Masai individuals of all ages and found that the coronary vessels of the Masai were just as atherosclerotic as those of US citizens, perhaps even more so. But severe sclerotic changes, so-called raised lesions, were rare; the sclerotic changes in the Masai were situated inside the vessel walls, leaving the inner surface of the vessels smooth. And in the 50 hearts he studied, there was no evidence that myocardial infarction had occurred in any of them.[19d]

Professor Mann thought that the Masai were protected from coronary heart disease by the size of their coronary arteries. These were much wider than those of most Western people, probably because the hearts of the Masai have worked hard while the men were running after the cattle. Many of the Masai tribesmen whom Mann examined were splendidly fit, as good as, or better than, superior sportsmen. It is no coincidence that some of the world's best runners come from Kenya.

Thus, it is possible to gorge on cholesterol and animal fat and still keep the blood cholesterol very low. The diet-heart idea should have been discarded after such evidence was published. The lessons learned from the studies of the Masai and Samburu present an insurmountable challenge to defenders of the diet-heart idea. But the idea is still flourishing, and nobody seems challenged. In fact, the Masai and the Samburu populations are not mentioned at all in official reviews of the diet-heart idea.

It is worth mentioning another interesting observation from Kenya. In that country there are many Indian emigrants. Although they all come from India, their diets are not similar. Non-Muslim Indians from Gujarat live on a lactovegetarian diet while Muslim Indians from Punjab eat eggs and meat, drink twice the amount of milk as their compatriots from Gujarat and never use vegetable oil. In other words, the non-Muslim Indians live as though they had been listening to the cholesterol campaign to avoid coronary heart disease, while the Muslims act as if they're doing all they can to have a heart attack. But the mortality rate from coronary heart disease is equal in both populations.[25]

A much larger aberration from the diet-heart idea comes from the studies of Dr. S. L. Malhotra of Bombay, India. Curiously, his work is never cited in the many reviews that call for a low-fat, "prudent" diet. He studied coronary heart disease among more than one million male employees of the Indian railways. During a five-year period, he recorded 679 deaths from heart disease. He noted that the highest rate of heart disease, 135 per 100,000 employees, occurred in Madras in southern India; the lowest rate, 20 per 100,000 employees, occurred in Punjab in northern India.

Thus, death from coronary heart disease occurred about

seven times more frequently in Madras, and those who died av-eraged twelve years younger than those in Punjab. But in Punjab, people ate ten to twenty times more fat and smoked eight times more cigarettes. And while the small amount of fat that people ate in the heart-disease-prone province of Madras was mainly of vegetable origin, the fat they gorged on in the Punjab was mainly of animal origin.[26]

Have patients with heart disease eaten more fat?

One way that scientists determine the causes of a disease is by performing a so-called case-control study. In a case-control study, scientists select a number of patients with the disease in question and a control group containing just as many people without the disease of the same age and sex and from the same geographic area. Then they ask how the patients differ from the controls. What do they do for a living? How much do they smoke and drink? What do they eat? Are they fatter or slimmer than the controls? What is the composition of their blood? Are they ex-posed more than the controls to environmental pollutants? The number of questions scientists can ask is limited only by their imagination and by the funds available.

In North Dakota, a case-control study was performed by Dr. William Zukel and his team. For one year, they studied all the men who had suffered symptoms of heart disease; for each case they chose two healthy men of the same age as controls. Dr. Zukel was especially interested in the diet of the participants during the month before the first symptoms or before the interview. If the interviewee had died, his wife or nearest relatives were ques-tioned.

Altogether 228 men had suffered symptoms of coronary dis-ease. Researchers obtained a detailed description of the diet from 162 of them. The conclusion of the study was that control indi-viduals were more likely to be manual workers, while the pa-tients were more likely to be smokers. But the diet did not differ between patients and control individuals; they ate the same amount of saturated and polyunsaturated fat and the same number of calories.[27]

In Ireland another group of researchers under the guidance of Dr. Aileen Finegan performed a similar investigation. For a whole year they studied the diet of 100 men who had suffered from a heart attack. The diet of these men was compared with that of 50 healthy men of the same age. Dr. Finegan and her team could not find any dietary differences either; the patients had eaten practically the same kind and amount of fats as the control individuals.[28]

A similar study—the Ireland-Boston study—was performed in a collaboration between researchers from Harvard University and the University of Dublin in Ireland under the guidance of Dr. Lawrence Kushi. The researchers selected men from Ireland who had brothers living in Boston for at least ten years. These two groups were compared with each other and with a third group of adult sons of Irish immigrants in Boston, a total of 1000 men. Now to the questions. How many would die from a heart attack during the next 20 years? And did their way of living differ from that of the others?

The researchers did not get a simple answer. Relatively speaking, more Boston brothers died from a heart attack than individuals from either of the other two groups, but the difference was so small that it could well have been due to chance. It could also have been due to the fact that the Boston brothers smoked more often and had higher blood pressure. The notion that their diet played an important role is unlikely because, contrary to the diet-heart idea, the men in Boston consumed less animal fat and less cholesterol than their brothers in Ireland, and more polyunsaturated oils than the immigrants' sons. And there was no difference between the blood cholesterol values of the three groups.[29] Yet, in spite of these negative findings, this study is often cited as strongly supportive of the diet-heart idea.[30]

More embarrassing data

Another "proof" of the diet-heart idea is a study performed in cooperation between the National Heart, Lung and Blood Institute and the University Hospital in Puerto Rico, conducted by Dr. Tavia Gordon. In Framingham, Puerto Rico and Honolulu, more than sixteen thousand healthy, middle-aged men were questioned about their dietary habits. Six years later the dietary habits of those who had suffered a heart attack were compared with the habits of those who had not. In Puerto Rico and Honolulu heart attack victims had consumed smaller amounts of starchy foods (such as bread, potatoes and rice) than the others; in Framingham they had eaten smaller amounts of "other carbohydrates." Eating starch or other carbohydrates should therefore protect against coronary heart disease, according to the authors of the report.

But the percentage of calories from starch did not differ between the healthy individuals and the patients except in Framingham, where those who had suffered a heart attack had eaten more starch than the others.

In Puerto Rico and in Honolulu, heart attack victims had consumed more polyunsaturated oils than those who had not had a heart attack. Although this observation is contrary to what was expected and thus most discouraging for those who advise people to consume more vegetable oils, the study authors did not mention this fact in the summary of their research.[31]

A similar study, led by Dr. Daniel McGee of the Framingham heart study, concerned 8000 Japanese immigrants in Hawaii. Researchers questioned them about their diet over a 24-hour period, and ten years later they compared the diet of those who had suffered a heart attack during the ten years with the diet of those who had not.

Those who had suffered a heart attack had eaten the same amount of animal fat and protein as the others but smaller amounts of carbohydrates. Ignoring these results, the authors recommended eating either more carbohydrates *or* less animal fat, as if the study had shown that either dietary modification would be effective. In the report summary, the authors failed to mention that the difference between the diets of both groups was not greater than what could have been produced by chance.[32]

Tabulating the results

By 1998, a total of 27 studies had been published including 34 groups (cohorts) of patients and control individuals and more than 150,000 individuals. In three of these 34 cohorts, patients with coronary disease had eaten more animal fat than the control individuals, and in one cohort they had eaten *less*. In the rest of the groups—30 in all—investigators found no difference in animal fat consumption between those who had heart disease and those who did not. In three cohorts the patients had eaten *more* polyunsaturated vegetable oils than the control individuals, and in only one they had eaten less.[33]

In the studies mentioned above, the researchers try to force the figures down into the cholesterol shoe, but neither heels nor toes will fit. According to some of the researchers, we should eat less saturated fat; according to others we should consume more polyunsaturated oils. Still others recommend carbohydrates or fiber or vegetables, depending on the haphazard results of the most recent investigation.

Why are the results of these studies so contradictory? One reason is that dietary information gleaned through questionnaires or interviews is unreliable; most of us simply cannot remember exactly what we ate a day ago. This is a valid objection that has been raised by many serious researchers. Nevertheless, the results of dietary recall studies are often used to support the diet-heart theory, even in the most prestigious reviews.

Even worse, researchers often draw conclusions from dietary recall studies when the results are not statistically significant. For example, the National Research Council published the following statement in *Diet and Health*: "Percentage of calories from SFAs [saturated fatty acids] was positively associated

THE MEDITERRANEAN DIET

Ancel Keys gained fame not only as the author of the Seven Countries study but also as the earliest proponent of the so-called Mediterranean Diet. "The heart of what we now consider the Mediterranean diet is mainly vegetarian," said Keys. "Pasta in many forms, leaves sprinkled with olive oil, all kinds of vegetables in season, and often cheese, all finished off with fruit and frequently washed down with wine." The diet of Italy and Greece, say the pundits, is low in animal foods with saturated fat contributing less than 8 percent of calories. Keys refers to saturated fat as "that dietary villain."

While the diet of Italy and Greece certainly contains bread and pasta, along with a variety of fruits and vegetables, anyone who has eaten in an Italian or Greek restaurant, traveled to the Mediterranean or looked at an Italian or Greek cookbook would conclude that these diets are certainly not vegetarian. Meat and fish are consumed every day by all but the poorest members of these societies; eggs are hidden in sauces, soups and casseroles; and sausages, meats, butter, cream and lard all provide abundant saturated fats.

And cheese consumption, especially in Greece, is very high. One food writer, who lived in Greece for many years, estimates that the peasants on Crete eat at least one-half pound of goat cheese per day. This would provide 600 calories or 25 percent of a 2400-calorie diet, just from cheese alone. Since the fat in goat cheese is almost 70 percent saturated, one-half pound of cheese per day would supply about 18 percent of calories as saturated fat. Other foods in the diet would bring the portion of saturated fat—"that dietary villain"—even higher.

Let us have a look at the consumption statistics that are available to us for five Mediterranean countries:

	1961-63 to 1983-85 Percent Change in Saturated Fat Consumption	1965-69 and 1991-92 Percent Change in CHD Mortality
Italy	+69	-61
Greece	+65	+13
Spain	+43	+10
Portugal	+10	-46
France	+28	-20

These figures show that Mediterranean people ate much more saturated fat in 1991-92 than 25 years earlier, but during the same period (with 5-6 years displacement) the number of heart attack deaths increased a little in only two of the countries; in the other three it *decreased*, and to a marked degree.

Data from 1986 *FAO Production Yearbook* 40, 1987; and *World Health Statistics Annual*, 1993.

with risk of CHD in the rural sample of the Puerto Rican and the Ireland-Boston studies."[34]

If you go to the library and look into the tables of these papers you will see that the differences found were not statistically significant, which means that the results were simply due to chance. And why didn't the authors of *Diet and Health* mention that, if anything, heart attack patients consumed *more* polyunsaturated fatty acids?

In a joint statement by the American Heart Association and the National Heart, Lung and Blood Institute, researchers declared: ". . . showing the link between diet and CHD, particularly impressive results [were produced in] the Western-Electric, the Honolulu Heart, the Zutphen and the Ireland-Boston studies."[35]

Yet the tables published in these studies showed that only in the Honolulu heart study had the patients eaten significantly more saturated fat. But they had also consumed significantly more polyunsaturated oils, just the opposite of what we have been led to expect.

Dietary cholesterol

For many years we have been told that we should not eat food containing too much cholesterol because cholesterol in our food makes cholesterol levels in our blood go up, and when cholesterol in our blood goes up, the heart is in danger. In particular, eggs have been singled out because egg yolk is richer in cholesterol than any other food. The fear of eggs has advanced to the point that researchers who study the influence of dietary cholesterol must ask the ethics committee of their university for approval if they want to give healthy people two eggs per day!

If cholesterol in our food causes heart disease, then CHD patients must logically have eaten more cholesterol than people who have no symptoms of heart disease.

But the research tells a different story. Table 1B lists data from studies that compared the consumption of cholesterol by healthy individuals and by CHD patients.

It is easy to see that there were no major differences between the two groups. In some of the studies, patients with heart disease had eaten a little more cholesterol than the control individuals, but in equally many studies, the control individuals had eaten a little more cholesterol than the CHD patients. In fact, the mean consumption of cholesterol in the CHD groups was 506 mg per day, slightly less than the mean cholesterol consumption of 518 mg per day in the control group. If the diet-heart idea were true, the mean cholesterol consumption in the CHD group would have been significantly higher than that of the controls.

Drawing conclusions

In summary, the most we can say for the many studies that

Table 1B. Comparison of the amount of cholesterol eaten per day by patients with coronary heart disease and age- and sex-matched control individuals in ten studies.

CHOLESTEROL EATEN PER DAY, IN MG

		Patients with CHD	Healthy Subjects
Male Chicago workers[36]		721	757
Framingham citizens[37]	men	708	716
	women	520	477
Puerto Rican men[38]	urban	449	442
	rural	335	358
Framingham citizens[39]		534	529
Puerto Ricans[39]		419	417
Honolulu citizens[39]		549	555
Honolulu citizens[40]		558	552
Men from Zutphen, The Netherlands[41]		446	429
Irish men from Ireland and the US[29]		854	832
Citizens from Rancho Bernardo, California, USA[42]	men	470	409
	women	226	309
Participants in the LRC study[43]			
	age 30-59	427	416
	age 60-79	423	355
Hawaiian citizens[44]	Hawaiian men	510	680
	Japanese men	466	587

have been performed to test the diet-heart hypothesis is that there is a weak association between the coronary mortality in various countries and the amount of fat available for them to eat, but *no* difference between the amount of fat eaten by coronary patients and by healthy individuals. Such discrepancies clearly indicate that the factor studied is not a causal one.

Another example is the association between prosperity and CHD. The mean income in various countries parallels the number of heart attacks; coronary heart disease is common in rich countries and usually rare in poor countries. But in rich countries poor people die more often from heart attacks than rich people.

Again, calories from animal food are more expensive than calories from vegetable food. Usually, the common denominator for countries where people eat lots of animal food is prosperity. In prosperous countries high-fat foods are abundant, but so are stress-provoking factors. In addition, more people smoke, fewer people perform manual labor, industrial pollution of the environment is most often worse and the ability to diagnose coronary heart disease is better. People in prosperous countries also live longer. Instead of dying from infectious diseases or malnutrition when they are young, they die from diseases related to old age, such as coronary heart disease. Any of these factors or their combination, or something else that I have not thought about, may explain why people die more often from a heart attack in prosperous countries than in poor ones.

Prosperity, high-fat foods and coronary heart disease thus go together. Statistical correlations may therefore arise when different countries are compared, especially if countries that do not follow the usual pattern are excluded. But inside the countries there is no correlation because it is not prosperity or high-fat foods in and of themselves that cause coronary disease.[45]

Soft science

In 1988 the US Surgeon General's Office decided to write

the "final and definitive" report on the dangers of dietary fat. The project did not go smoothly, however, and eleven years later a letter was circulated in the Office explaining that the report would be cancelled. "The report was initiated with a preconceived opinion of the conclusions," admitted Bill Harlan, associate director of the Office of Disease Prevention at National Institutes of Health and a member of the oversight committee. "But the science behind those opinions was not holding up." There was no other public announcement, however, and no press release about these revolutionary conclusions.

Harlan's statement was given to Gary Taubes, an American science journalist with many international awards for his articles, most of them aimed at exposing poor and deficient science. He has examined the basis for the current dietary advice on fats and oils by interviewing hundreds of researchers and civil servants, reading thousands of government reports and transcriptions of congressional hearings and by studying the scientific literature in depth. The result was an article entitled "The Soft Science of Dietary Fat" published in the prestigious *Science Magazine*.[46]

Taubes described the manoeuvres of the Senate Select Committee on Nutrition and Human Needs, founded in 1968 and chaired by Senator George McGovern. The Committee had a mandate to eradicate malnutrition in the US. Two young lawyers who had been influenced by a few researchers with extreme views on dietary fat decided to also address the question of *over*nutrition in America. At that time it appeared evident that high-fat food, especially food high in animal fat, was the main cause of coronary heart disease. Although the Committee received volumes of testimony that contradicted these extreme views, its members were committed to the diet-heart idea and believed that the people should be taught.

The Committee's task of researching and writing the first "Dietary Goals for the United States" was assigned to Nick Mottern, a political journalist without any scientific background and no experience in writing about science. To avoid the scientific and medical controversy, he relied almost exclusively on nutritionist Mark Hegsted, from the Harvard School of Public Health, who happened to be a categorical believer in the diet-heart idea.

The final Committee report, the so-called McGovern Report, promoted the same recommendations as those of the American Heart Association. It was violently criticized by many researchers and, for obvious reasons, by the dairy, egg and cattle industries. It was therefore easy for the authors to defend the report. Animal fat was just as dangerous as cigarettes, they said, and to argue against the report proved that the opponents were either hopelessly out of date, or paid by the food industry.

Robert Levy, director of the NHLBI, found his position awkward. "The good senators came out with the guidelines and then called us in to get advice." The politicians, the press and public opinion had already bought the idea about the dangers of animal fat—now it was up to researchers to follow with the science. Those who are familiar with the medical literature know that they listened.

How did the cholesterol establishment react to Gary Taubes' exposé? Here are three quotations from a critical letter[47] sent to *Science Magazine* by Professor Scott Grundy, one of the leading proponents of the diet-heart idea.

"The significance of saturated fatty acids has been demonstrated by an enormous number of high-quality studies carried out with dietary fat in the fields of animal research, epidemiology, metabolism and clinical trials."

"Several trials reveal that substitution of unsaturated fatty acids for saturated fatty acids lowers the incidence of CHD."

If you have read this chapter from the beginning you will know that the two first allegations are very far from the truth. But what about the third quotation?

"Evidence is abundant that elevated LDL is a major cause of CHD and that lowering serum LDL levels reduces CHD risk."

If you think this is true. . . read on.

Myth 2

High Cholesterol Causes Heart Disease

*In our need to understand, to explain, and to treat, the tempta-
tion to impute causality to association is pervasive and hard to
resist. It is the most important reason for error in medicine.*

Petr Skrabanek
James McCormick
(Authors of *Follies and Fallacies in Medicine*)

Large and small percentages

Framingham is a small town near Boston, Massachusetts.
Since the early 1950s a large number of Framingham citizens
has taken part in a study surveying all the factors that may play
a role in the development of atherosclerosis and heart disease.
Among other things their cholesterol was measured frequently.[1]

After five years the researchers made an observation that
has become one of the cornerstones of the diet-heart idea. When
they divided the participants into three groups having low, me-
dium and high cholesterol values, they observed that in the latter group more had died from a heart attack than in the two
other groups. A high cholesterol level predicted a greater risk of
a heart attack, they said; high cholesterol is a risk factor for
coronary heart disease.

The predictive value of blood cholesterol levels was confirmed in the greatest medical experiment in history, the Multiple Risk Factor Intervention Trial, also called MRFIT. In that trial researchers measured the blood cholesterol of more than 300,000 American middle-aged men.

Six years later professor Jeremiah Stamler, the director of MRFIT, and his co-workers from Chicago asked how many of these men, the so-called "screenees" (see page 49) had died and why.[2] The participants were divided into ten groups of equal size, so-called deciles, according to their cholesterol values. The first decile thus consisted of the tenth of the men with the lowest cholesterol values, and the tenth decile consisted of those with the highest cholesterol values.[3]

The researchers' analysis showed that in the tenth decile, four times more men had died of a heart attack than in the first decile. Professor Stamler's team put it another way: The risk of dying from a heart attack with cholesterol above 265 was 413 percent greater than with cholesterol below 170.

Four hundred and thirteen percent! How frightening! But let us look at the real figures, not just at the percentages. With statistics you can change black to white, or vice versa, as any politician will tell you.

How many men in the MRFIT study had, in fact, died of a heart attack? The total number was 2258, or 0.6 percent of the more than 300,000 men investigated. You could also say that 99.4 percent did not die from a heart attack.

Four hundred ninety four of those with the highest cholesterol value (the tenth decile), or 1.3 percent, died from a heart attack. We could also describe these results by saying that 98.7 percent of those with the very highest cholesterol values were alive after six years.

Among those with the lowest values, the first decile, 95 men, or 0.3 percent, died from a heart attack, while the rest, 99.7 percent, survived. Thus, the difference in numbers of deaths between the first and the tenth decile was only one percentage point

"THE MOST EXACT DATA BASE" - THE SCREENEES OF MRFIT

The figures from the MRFIT study included both the 12,000 participating men, but also the more than 300,000 men who were excluded for various reasons. A large number of studies concerning the follow-up of these screenees has been published in well-known international medical journals, and these studies are cited again and again as the strongest proof that there is a linear association between blood cholesterol concentrations and the risk of future heart disease. (Most researchers have found that cholesterol is significant only above a certain level.)

Unfortunately, the data presented in the MRFIT reports have been carelessly produced. In a systematic search of the literature on the MRFIT study, Professor Lars Werkö, then director of the Swedish Council on Technology Assessment in Health Care, an independent governmental agency known for its integrity, found 34 papers reporting the relationship between serum cholesterol and mortality. He asked himself whether it really was necessary to publish all these reports as their results were so similar. "Have the editors really judged the original scientific value of each of these similar articles and deemed them worthy of publication? Or have they been impressed by the status of the research groups that authored these repetitive manuscripts, with the prestigious National Heart, Lung and Blood Institute in the background, and found that they have to succumb to the authorities?"

Worse than being repetitive, the data were inconsistent and highly questionable. For instance, the number of screenees varied greatly between the studies, from 316,099 to 361,266. In particular, Professor Werkö was critical of the studies reporting how many had died and why, because it is highly unlikely that all of 361,266 individuals could have been tracked after 6-12 years.

How the cause of death had been established was not reported but we can be rather confident that most of the reported causes were based on death certificates written by general practitioners. Not only is the information from death certificates highly unreliable (see pages 17-21), but, in many cases (between 6 and 20 percent, depending on the report), death certificates were actually missing. Yet some of the reports gave a detailed list of diagnoses for almost all deaths.

Furthermore, during the initial screening it came to light that one of the participating centers had falsified its data to increase the number of participants in the trial, possibly in order to obtain more financial support from the National Institutes of Health. This embarrassing matter received little mention in the follow-up reports, nor did the study authors mention the possibility that data falsification could have occurred in other centers as well. Instead, all discussion of the issue of quality control was studiously avoided. Wrote Professor Werkö: "In the many publications regarding the MRFIT screenees, it is obvious that the authors are more interested in the mathematical treatment of large figures than in the quality of these figures or how they were obtained."

In spite of all these irregularities, the follow-up reports on the MRFIT screenees are still cited as "the most exact database regarding the relation of risk factors to mortality in the healthy male US population."

Werkö L. Analysis of the MRFIT screenees: a methodological study. *Journal of Internal Medicine* 237, 507-518, 1995

(99.7 percent minus 98.7 percent).

One percentage point doesn't have the same alarming effect as Dr. Stamler's 413 percent, but both figures are correct because 1.3 is 413 percent of 0.3.

The excess of deaths was most pronounced in the tenth decile, which included, it should be remembered, almost all individuals with the rare, inherited disease called familial hyper-cholesterolemia. These people have considerably higher choles-terol values than normal individuals, and they often have severe atherosclerosis and cardiovascular disease in early life. A little less than one percent of humanity has familial hypercholesterol-emia or some other kind of genetic problem that interferes with fat metabolism. This means that about ten percent of the tenth decile (10 times 1 percent) were abnormal in this respect. Thus, in a complicated way, the statistics demonstrated what we al-ready knew—that patients with an inborn error of cholesterol metabolism have a greater risk of dying from heart disease. (For more about MRFIT, see Chapter 6.)

There are more ways that risk factor statistics can be used to magnify trivial differences. Let us go back to the Framingham study.

Great or small differences?

To illustrate the association between blood cholesterol and the risk of dying from a heart attack, the researchers from Framingham constructed an interesting graph, shown in Fig-ure 2A.[4] Two bell-shaped curves are seen. The horizontal axis, or x-axis, represents levels of blood cholesterol while the ver-tical or y-axis concerns the number of individuals measured.

The curves in Figure 2A are called Gaussian or "bell" curves. When plotted in a diagram like Figure 2A, all mea-surements in biology usually produce a Gaussian curve with a distinctive parabolic or bell shape that rises slowly at first from the baseline on each side and then rapidly increases in slope at the center. The total area under the curve gives the number of individuals investigated. If, for example, you graph the heights of a random number of people, short individuals will be situated in the area beneath the curve's left slope and tall individuals will be situated in the area beneath its right slope. When a bell curve is symmetrical, the mean value of the group lies at the top of the curve.

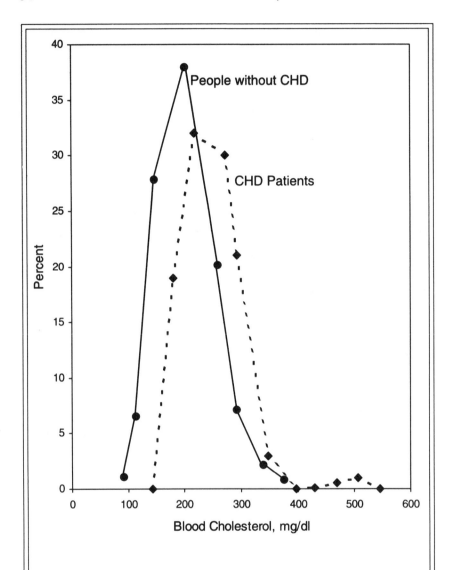

Figure 2A. The distribution of the participants in the Framingham project according to their blood cholesterol. The solid line represents 1378 individuals without coronary disease; the broken line represents 193 patients with coronary disease. Data from Kannel, Castelli and Gordon.[4]

Let's take a careful look at Figure 2A. The broken line represents the cholesterol levels of all middle-aged men in the Framingham study who, sixteen years after the start of the project, had suffered a heart attack. The unbroken line represents the cholesterol levels of the men who had not. The first group consisted of 193 individuals, the other of 1378. The second group is eight times larger but the area under the two curves is almost equal. This is because the vertical y-axis does not represent the number of individuals tested, as is customary, but the percentage of the total at each blood cholesterol point. Thus, for example, about 32 percent of CHD patients had cholesterol levels around 220 mg/dl while about 38 percent of non-CHD patients had cholesterol levels around 220 mg/dl.

The curve for the CHD patients is slightly asymmetrical and has a little hump far to the right, which represents those with familial hypercholesterolemia. Otherwise, the two curves appear identical except that the curve of the coronary patients is placed a little to the right; their cholesterol values are approximately 5-10 percent higher than the values of those who remained free of cardiovascular disease.

Most people probably think that those who have a heart attack almost always have large amounts of cholesterol in their blood. The curves demonstrate, however, that the difference is marginal. In fact, the graph shows that almost half of those who had a heart attack had low cholesterol.

Proponents of the diet-heart idea allege that this small difference in blood cholesterol is one of the most important causes of atherosclerosis and coronary heart disease. But as we shall see, the difference may be due to several other factors.

No risk after forty-seven
Thirty years after the first cholesterol measurements in Framingham, the researchers again asked themselves what

had happened.[5] This time, a few more of those with high cholesterol levels had died. I use the word *few* for a reason. On average one percent of all men with high cholesterol died each year during the 30 follow-up years. During the first ten years, about a quarter of one percent of the total died each year. As time passed, the percentage that died each year naturally grew larger and larger. Among those with the lowest cholesterol values, only half as many died; and, as in almost all earlier investigations, women with low cholesterol died equally often as did women with high cholesterol.

But these figures concerned *all* causes of death. The researchers said nothing about death from heart disease! And heart mortality was the main issue of the whole project. We are entitled to ask just why the Framingham investigators "forgot" to tell us about it.

Now to the most interesting point, illustrated in Figure 2B. For men above age 47, cholesterol levels made no difference. Those who had low cholesterol at the age of 48 died just as often as those with high cholesterol!

Thus, the Framingham study showed that if you reach age 47, it doesn't matter whether your cholesterol is high or low! I have never met any believer in the diet-heart idea who has even raised an eyebrow when confronted with this astounding fact.

Blood cholesterol is usually at its highest level at about the age of fifty. It is after this age that heart attacks usually appear, increasing in frequency year by year. After age fifty, atherosclerosis also accelerates, but the first signs of atherosclerosis in the artery wall appear much earlier, between the ages of 20 and 30.

Atherosclerotic lesions are a kind of inflammation involving the smooth muscle cells and elastic fibers of the arteries as well as the white blood cells. In the early stages, cholesterol may not be present at all and the lesions do not, in general, impede blood flow. Much later, usually after age 50, chole-

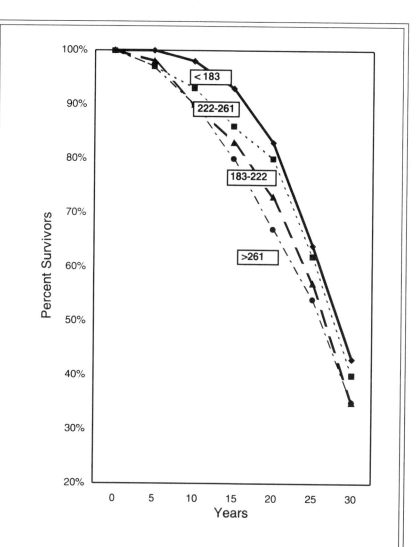

Figure 2B. Survival curves for men between age 48 and age 57 in the Framingham study. The men are divided into four groups according to their blood cholesterol value. Note that the curve for those with a blood cholesterol between 183 and 222 is situated below the curve for those with a blood cholesterol between 222 and 261; the latter thus lived longer than those with lower cholesterol. Data from Anderson, Castelli and Levy.[5]

sterol and various lipids may be deposited in these lesions, causing them to thicken irregularly and to protrude into the interior of the vessels. It is these so-called raised lesions that are dangerous because they block the passage of blood through the arteries.

With these facts in mind, how do you explain the findings that high cholesterol seems to be dangerous at the age of 30, but not after 47? If high cholesterol produces raised lesions because its level in the blood is a little higher than usual, why is high cholesterol a risk factor at the age of 30, when cholesterol is rarely found in the atherosclerotic lesions and raised lesions are rare, but not after 47, the period of life when cholesterol is likely to build up in the blood vessels?

Furthermore, few die from a heart attack before the age of 48, and most of those who do die are diabetics or have a rare genetic problem. More than 95 percent of all heart attacks occur in people older than 48. If cholesterol has importance only for the very few who have a heart attack before 48, why should the rest of us worry at all about blood cholesterol levels and high-fat food?

The Framingham findings are not a rare exception. High cholesterol has no importance in Australian men above age 74 either, according to a study by Dr. L. A. Simons and his co-workers at St. Vincent's Hospital in Sydney, Australia.[6] Similar findings were uncovered in a study by Dr. Peter Zimetbaum and his co-workers at the Albert Einstein College of Medicine in the Bronx, NY.[7] They found that neither total nor LDL-cholesterol predicted the risk of having a heart attack or any other cardiovascular disease in very old men. Curiously, the authors concluded that "the findings of this study suggest that an unfavorable lipoprotein profile increases the risk for cardiovascular morbidity and mortality."

Unfortunately, this happens all too frequently. Researchers get a result that is contrary to the cholesterol hypotheses, and yet they write conclusions indicating that their findings are in support. These misleading conclusions are most often written up in the summary of the papers, the only part of the paper that most doctors and researchers are likely to read. To find the contradictory results, you have to read the whole paper and meticulously study the tables.

In the elderly, high cholesterol even seems to be protective. This was the surprising finding of Dr. Harlan Krumholz and his co-workers at the Department of Cardiovascular Medicine at Yale University. They followed 997 elderly men and women living in the Bronx, NY. During a four-year period, about twice as many of the individuals with low cholesterol had a heart attack or died from one compared to those with the highest cholesterol levels.[8]

Let me return to the study of the Framingham group. Perhaps you think that the cholesterol campaign was cancelled after the results of the Framingham study came in. Not at all. The reason low cholesterol levels were associated with greater mortality, said the investigators, was that people with low cholesterol levels were dying of other diseases. But their results contradicted that explanation. Wrote the authors: Those whose cholesterol had *decreased* by itself during these 30 years ran a greater risk of dying than those whose cholesterol had *increased*. To cite the report: "For each 1% mg/dl drop of cholesterol there was an 11 percent increase in coronary and total mortality."

Thus, not only total mortality but also coronary mortality had increased.

Now, stop for a moment! For many years we have been told how important it is to lower our cholesterol to prevent coronary heart disease. But the Framingham study demonstrated that if blood cholesterol *decreases* by itself, the risk of dying *increases*.

Few people know about this alarming finding, and the study is rarely discussed in medical reviews on cholesterol and heart disease. Even worse, when the study is noted, it is cited as *supporting* the diet-heart idea! Consider the joint statement by the American Heart Association and the National Heart, Lung and Blood Institute in their review titled *The Cholesterol Facts*: "The results of the Framingham study indicate that a 1% reduction . . . of cholesterol [corresponds to a] 2% reduction in CHD risk".[9]

Please go back to the citation from the report. Yes, you are right. According to the original report, mortality *increased*, and by 11 percent for each 1 mg/dl reduction in blood cholesterol. But the review stated that mortality *decreased*.

Your next thought might be that the distinguished authors of the review were referring to another of the numerous reports from Framingham, but that is not the case. And, as we shall see, this was only one of many "mistakes." For example, in 1987, the Framingham authors published a new report concerning the 30 years of follow-up in Framingham.[10] Without presenting anything other than complicated ratios and statistical calculations, and without referring to their previous report, they stated: "The most important overall finding is the emergence of the total cholesterol concentration as a risk factor for CHD in the elderly."

Isn't it strange that the cholesterol liner continues its voyage without any reactions from the passengers or crew? The few who have observed that the ship is leaning are numbed by the captain's assurances that it has only struck an iceberg.[11]

Rule with many exceptions

Most supporters of the diet-heart idea think that the increased risk of coronary heart disease is present at all cholesterol levels. Those who have a cholesterol level of 200 mg/dl, for example, are worse off than those with a cholesterol level of 150 mg/dl; and those who have a cholesterol level of 250 mg/dl are at even greater risk. The pharmaceutical companies love this concept for it implies that almost everyone should be treated, even those with normal cholesterol levels.

The truth, were it known, would send pharmaceutical stocks plunging. In most studies, the increased risk is present only above a level of cholesterol that includes just a small percentage of the total population.[12] And women can stop worrying immediately because most studies have found that high cholesterol is not a risk factor for the female sex. Few comments have been made on this peculiar fact in all the vast literature on cholesterol. When it is mentioned at all, it is said that female sex hormones protect against heart attacks.

In fact, it seems more dangerous for women to have low cholesterol than high. Dr. Bernard Forette and a team of French researchers from Paris found that old women with very high cholesterol live the longest. The death rate was more than five times higher for women who had very low cholesterol. In their report, the French doctors warned against cholesterol lowering in elderly women,[13] but they could as well have warned against cholesterol lowering in any woman or, to be more precise, in anyone at all.

At a workshop held at the National Heart, Lung and Blood Institute, researchers looked at every study that had been published about the risk of having high or low cholesterol and came to the same conclusion: Mortality was higher for women with low cholesterol than for women with high cholesterol.[14] We'll return to this subject in Chapter 7.

Another finding that should cause some discomfort among diet-heart proponents is that whereas high cholesterol has a slight association with increased risk for men in the US, it has no such association for men in Canada. This conclusion was reached by Dr. Gilles Dagenais and his team in Quebec after having followed almost 5000 healthy middle-aged men for 12 years.[15] They explained away their surprising finding by assuming that more than 12 years were needed to see the harmful effects of high cholesterol levels; obviously they were ignorant of the Framingham 30-year follow-up study results.

Neither is blood cholesterol important for those who have

already had a heart attack. For instance, Dr. Henry Shanoff and his team at the University Hospital of Toronto studied 120 men ten years after their recovery from a heart attack and found that those with low cholesterol had a second coronary just as often as those with high cholesterol.[16] Many others have confirmed their findings.[17]

In Sweden, Professors Lars-Erik Böttiger and Lars A. Carlson at the Karolinska Hospital found that the risk of coronary heart disease was higher for men with the highest cholesterol, but the risk was considerably lower than in Framingham.[18] They also found that if all kinds of vascular disease caused by atherosclerosis were considered, the risk was not increased at all. Those with low cholesterol died from heart disease just as often as those with high cholesterol.[19]

And there are more exceptions, such as the Maori, Polynesians who migrated to New Zealand several hundred years ago. Unlike the native Polynesians, Maoris often die from heart attacks, but they do so whether their cholesterol is low or high.[20]

In Russia, *low* cholesterol is associated with increased risk of coronary heart disease. This was the surprising finding of Dr. Dmitri Shestov from the Russian Academy of Medical Sciences in St. Petersburg. Dr. Shestov and his colleagues, one of whom was Professor Herman Tyroler from the Department of Epidemiology at the University of North Carolina, also analyzed HDL- and LDL-cholesterol, the so-called "good" and "bad" cholesterol. (More on HDL and LDL later.) High levels of LDL are supposed to make us prone to heart disease, but the investigators found that *low* levels of LDL-cholesterol were associated with increased risk; and this increased risk was not due to low levels of HDL-cholesterol, the good guy. In fact, those with low LDL values had the highest HDL values.[21]

Thus, high cholesterol is said to be dangerous for Americans but not for Canadians, Stockholmers, Russians or Maoris. High cholesterol is said to be dangerous for men, but not for women; it is said to be dangerous for healthy men, but not for coronary patients; and it is said to be dangerous for men of 30, but not for those of 48. And high cholesterol may even be beneficial for older people. Such discrepancies indicate that the association between high cholesterol and coronary heart disease is not due to simple cause and effect. The most likely interpretation is that high cholesterol is not dangerous in itself but a marker for something else.

Many scientists who are critical of the diet-heart idea still have the impression that an increased level of cholesterol in the blood may be dangerous just because of its *association* with coronary mortality. Few scientists realize that the association is unsystematic and weak. And even if the association were both systematic and strong, this would not prove that it is the high cholesterol level itself that causes atherosclerosis or heart disease. There are at least five other plausible explanations for higher cholesterol levels in patients with coronary heart disease.

Guilt by association

Familial hypercholesterolemia is one of them. Individuals suffering from this disease run a greater risk of dying early from a heart attack, and they also have significantly raised cholesterol levels. It is accepted dogma that high cholesterol levels, by promoting atherosclerosis, are the direct cause of their troubles. But, as I shall discuss later, the vascular changes seen in familial hypercholesterolemia are not the same as those of atherosclerosis.

Smoking generates a slight increase in blood cholesterol[22] but may induce heart disease by several other mechanisms, such as the production of free radicals. (See Chapter 7.) Thus smoking may induce a heart attack *and* elevated cholesterol.

Being overweight increases blood cholesterol a little, and weight reduction lowers it a little. Excess weight may cause heart disease because it means an excess burden to the heart.

FAMILIAL HYPERCHOLESTEROLEMIA - NOT AS RISKY AS YOU MAY THINK

Many doctors believe that most patients with familial hyper-cholesterolemia (FH) die from CHD at a young age. Obviously, they do not know the surprising finding of the Scientific Steering Committee at the Department of Public Health and Primary Care at Ratcliffe Infirmary in Oxford, England. For several years, these researchers followed more than 500 FH patients between the ages of 20 and 74 and compared patient mortality during this period with that of the general population.

During a three- to four-year period, six of 214 FH patients below age 40 died from CHD. This may not seem particularly frightening but as it is rare to die from CHD before the age of 40, the risk for these FH patients was almost 100 times that of the general population.

During a four- to five-year period, eight of 237 FH patients between ages 40 and 59 died, which was five times more than the general population. But during a similar period of time, only one of 75 FH patients between the ages of 60 and 74 died from CHD, when the expected number was two.

If these results are typical for FH, you could say that between ages 20 and 59, about 3 percent of the patients die from CHD, and between ages 60 and 74, less than 2 percent die, in both cases during a period of 3-4 years. The authors stressed that the patients had been referred because of a personal or family history of premature vascular disease and therefore were at a particularly high risk for CHD. Most patients with FH in the general population are unrecognized and untreated. Had the patients studied been representative for all FH patients, their prognosis would probably have been even better.

This view was recently confirmed by Dr. Eric Sijbrands and his coworkers from various medical departments in Amsterdam and Leiden, Netherlands. Out of a large group they found three individuals with very high cholesterol. A genetic analysis confirmed the diagnosis of FH and by tracing their family members backward in time, they came up with a total of 412 individuals. The coronary and total mortality of these members were compared with the mortality of the general Dutch population.

The striking finding was that those who lived during the 19th and early 20th century had normal mortality and lived a normal life span. In fact, those living in the 19th century had a *lower* mortality than the general population. After 1915 the mortality rose to a maximum between 1935 and 1964, but even at the peak, mortality was less than twice as high as in the general population.

Again, very high cholesterol levels alone do not lead to a heart attack. In fact, high cholesterol may even be protective against other diseases. This was the conclusion of Dr. Sijbrands and his colleagues. As support they cited the fact that genetically modified mice with high cholesterol are protected against severe bacterial infections.

"Doctor, don't be afraid because of my high cholesterol." These were the words of a 36-year-old lawyer who visited me for the first time for a health examination. And indeed, his cholesterol was high, over 400 mg/dl.

"My father's cholesterol was even higher," he added. "But he lived happily until he died at age 79 from cancer. And his brother, who also had FH, died at age 83. None of them ever complained of any heart problems." My "patient" is now 53, his brother is 56 and his cousin 61. All of them have extremely high cholesterol values, but none of them has any heart troubles, and none of them has ever taken cholesterol-lowering drugs.

So, if you happen to have FH, don't be too anxious. Your chances of surviving are pretty good, even surviving to old age.

Scientific Steering Committee on behalf of the Simon Broome Register Group. Risk of fatal coronary heart disease in familial hypercholesterolaemia. *British Medical Journal* 303, 893-896, 1991; Sijbrands EJG and others. Mortality over two centuries in large pedigree with familial hypercholesterolaemia: family tree mortality study. British Medical Journal 322, 1019-1023, 2001.

Excess weight also predisposes individuals to diabetes, another vascular disease that may cause CHD. Thus excess weight may induce CHD *and* elevated cholesterol.[23]

High blood pressure is also associated with high blood cholesterol. Hypertension, both untreated and treated, is seen in about one-third of all individuals with cholesterol levels above 260 mg/dl but only in 15-20 percent of those with cholesterol lower than 220 mg/dl.[24] High blood pressure or one of its underlying causes, such as stress, may provoke a heart attack *and* raise blood cholesterol.

In fact, it is stress, particularly emotional stress, that seems to cause the steepest rise in cholesterol. An academic exam, blood sampling or surgery, conflicts at work or at home, loss of a spouse or close friend and various types of performance demands have been found to increase cholesterol levels rapidly by 10 to 50 percent.[25] One explanation may be that during stress more cholesterol is produced by the liver and the adrenal glands because the body uses cholesterol to manufacture a variety of stress hormones. Thus, psychological stress may provoke a heart attack (for instance by a spasm of the coronary vessels) *and* an elevated cholesterol level.

That high cholesterol is a risk factor for heart disease may thus have many explanations, but none of them is ever discussed in the papers written by the proponents of the diet-heart idea.

"Look at Finland and Japan"

Perhaps you are wondering why Western people have such a morbid fear of heart disease when dying from a heart attack may not be too bad compared to the alternatives. After all, most of us would prefer to die quickly, without spending many years in a nursing home, crippled or senile. And remember that coronary heart disease is a disease of old age. In fact, on average, those who die from a heart attack have lived just as long as other people. Nevertheless, studies claiming an association in various countries between the average blood cholesterol levels and death rates from coronary disease are frequently used to justify the diet-heart idea. Let's look at some of the studies.

The most famous one is the Seven Countries study by Dr. Ancel Keys (see page 25) in which Keys pointed to an association between blood cholesterol and heart mortality in seven countries. "The correlation is obvious," wrote Dr. Keys. He illustrated his words with a graph.

It is not apparent from Dr. Keys' paper how he constructed his graph, but it is possible to draw a graph oneself by using the numbers from his tables. I have drawn such a graph, shown in Figure 2C, using the "hard" data, meaning average cholesterol values in various localities and the number who died from coronary heart disease ("CHD deaths per 10,000 in five years among CHD-free men"). If the diet-heart idea is correct, heart attacks should, of course, be consistently rare in areas where cholesterol levels are low and common where they are high. But as seen from my graph, in several countries some provinces had widely differing rates of heart disease, even though average blood cholesterol values were the same. Oddly, this important chart is not included in Dr. Keys' paper, although his paper is loaded with more or less relevant graphs.

If Keys had found a good correlation between cholesterol levels and heart disease, the points on the graph would have been located on or very near an upward diagonal line beginning at the intersection of the x- and y-axes. Instead, there is a notable "scattering" of the points in the chart. Note, for instance, that in the area of the graph where fatal heart attacks were less than 100 per 10,000, the cholesterol levels vary between the lowest and the second highest value.

It is difficult to conclude from Figure 2C that the number of heart disease deaths and levels of blood cholesterol are related. They may be statistically related, but we should be skeptical about correlations that depend on just one or two observations.

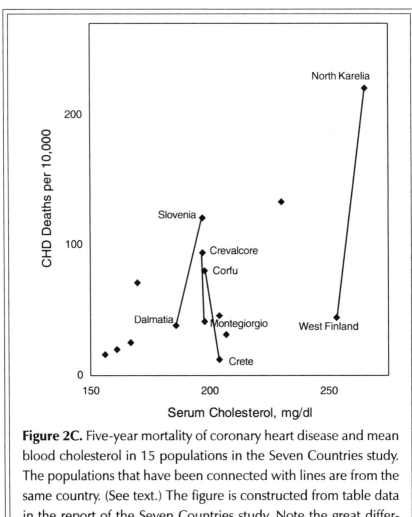

Figure 2C. Five-year mortality of coronary heart disease and mean blood cholesterol in 15 populations in the Seven Countries study. The populations that have been connected with lines are from the same country. (See text.) The figure is constructed from table data in the report of the Seven Countries study. Note the great differences in coronary mortality at similar blood cholesterol levels. Data from Keys, reference 10, Chapter 1.

For instance, cover the point labeled North Karelia with your hand and the slight impression of an association disappears completely.

The impression of association also disappears if you look at each country individually. I have drawn lines connecting districts located within the same country. Note that in Crevalcore,

Italy, the number of deaths from heart disease was 2.5 times greater than in Montegiorgio, Italy, although the average blood cholesterol was identical. In Slavonia, three times more died from heart disease than in Dalmatia, although the mean cholesterol in Slavonia was only insignificantly higher. In Finland, people living in North Karelia died five times more often from a heart attack than people living in the area of Turku although blood cholesterol differed only by a small amount. And, finally, on the Greek island of Corfu, people died five times more often from a heart attack than on nearby Crete, although their cholesterol was lower. The differences between the total number of heart attacks, fatal and nonfatal, were even larger.

Dr. Keys' data reveals another surprising finding: No correlation was found between diet and the major electrocardiographic findings recorded at the beginning of the study. Again, this finding appears only if you go to the tables of the study; it does not appear in the text or the figures. Considering that all electrocardiograms were analyzed in the American study center by specialists, this finding should carry more weight than the correlation with the clinical diagnosis or the diagnosis on the death certificate. Death certificates are far less reliable than electrocardiograms because they are written on location by various physicians with different diagnostic habits and varying degrees of competence.

In spite of the data in his tables, Dr. Keys concluded that the only factor that could explain the great differences between the number of heart attacks in the sixteen areas he analyzed was blood cholesterol levels. In particular, he stressed the low heart-disease mortality and lower cholesterol in Japan and the opposite findings in Finland.

Although the Seven Countries study flatly contradicts the diet-heart idea, proponents continually refer to is as proof. Their mantra: "Look at Finland and Japan."[26]

Let's look at Figure 2C once again. Eager to prove his hypothesis, Dr. Keys unintentionally covered up one of the most

MEASURING RELATIONSHIPS

In statistical methodology, the strength of an association between two variables—such as height and weight, or cholesterol levels and heart disease—is expressed by the correlation coefficient r.

When r is close to 1, an individual with a high value for one variable will likely have a high value for the other, and an individual with a low value for one variable will likely have a low value for the other. We say that there is a strong positive association between X and Y. When plotted on a graph, the individual points tend to cluster on either side of an ascending straight line or curve. In other words, the data make a "good fit."

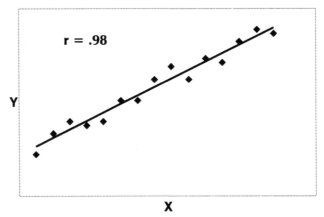

Example of a Strong, Positive Correlation Between X and Y

When r is close to -1, then an individual with a high value for one variable will likely have a low variable for the other. We say that there is a strong negative association between X and Y. When plotted on a graph, the individual points tend to cluster on either side of a descending line or curve. Once again, the data make a "good fit."

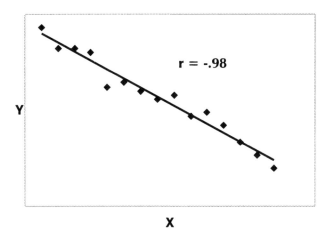

r = -.98

Example of a Strong, Negative Correlation Between X and Y

If r is close to zero, the points will be scattered randomly like the "starry sky," seen below.

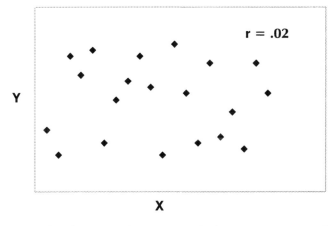

r = .02

Example of a Nonexistent Correlation Between X and Y

It must always be kept in mind that even though two variables X and Y show a strong association, that does not mean that a high X causes Y or, in case the correlation is inverse, that a low X causes Y.

interesting tracks. It is almost heartbreaking. I suspect that many of you have already asked the question that Dr. Keys had the opportunity to answer 30 years ago. It is doubtful that circumstances would allow us to answer it today. But, to ask it anyway, what is the factor that protects the inhabitants of Dalmatia, Montegiorgio, Turku and Crete from coronary heart disease that is lacking in Slavonia, Crevalcore, North Karelia and on Corfu?

Or, to turn the question around: Why does death from coronary heart disease occur three to five times more often in the latter areas? We can blame none of the well-known risk factors because Dr. Keys found that they were equally present in each pair of areas. If Dr. Keys and his co-workers had concentrated all their efforts in these eight places, if they had observed, investigated, questioned and turned over every stone, they might have found something helpful to mankind.

This is the most tragic aspect of the cholesterol folly. Interesting side tracks are left unexplored, observations that do not fit with the idea are put aside, and any opportunity for a discovery is allowed to slip by.

Or is it possible that Dr. Keys is right, only he studied too few countries? An association may be so weak that you have to make many observations to uncover it. Perhaps the correlation will appear if we study 27 countries instead of only seven? Let us see.

MONICA

For many years, the World Health Organization (WHO) has conducted a gigantic, international project on cardiovascular disease. Called MONICA, for "MONItoring of trends and determinants in CArdiovascular disease," the project was initially headed by the Chicago professor Dr. Jeremiah Stamler, one of the staunchest diet-heart proponents. One hundred thirteen groups of scientists and doctors in 27 countries throughout North America, Europe, Asia and Australia stud-

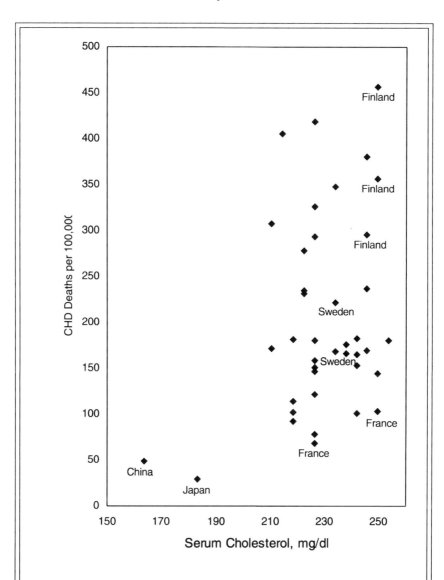

Figure 2D. The relationship between blood cholesterol and mortality in coronary heart disease according to data from the MONICA project. Note the great variations in coronary mortality at the same blood cholesterol levels. Data from Shanoff, Little and Csima.[16]

ied everything they thought could possibly be of importance for the development of cardiovascular disease, including, of course, the relationship between cholesterol levels and coronary mortality.[27]

The authors of this study have not yet published complete analyses of their data, even though the figures have been available for several years. But we can use their raw data to draw our own conclusions, as shown in Figure 2D.

The results are similar to those obtained from Dr. Keys' data (Figure 2C). The highest mortality is five times greater than the lowest one at the same level of blood cholesterol. In North Karelia mean blood cholesterol was 245 mg/dl with deaths from coronary heart disease at 493 per 100,000 inhabitants each year. In Fribourg, France, average blood cholesterol was also 245 mg/dl, but coronary mortality was only 102 per 100,000 inhabitants per year, only about a fifth.

Low mortality and high mean cholesterol values were noted in all the French locations. This is the so-called French Paradox. To explain the French Paradox, researchers cite factors considered representative of the Mediterranean diet—for instance, wine drinking and the use of olive oil instead of butter—as protection against coronary disease.

Actually, there is no French Paradox. A paradox implies that all other observations were in line with the diet-heart idea but, as you can see from Figure 2D, they were not. The French observations happened to be those that were most deviant, but high cholesterol and low coronary mortality were also observed in Augsburg, Germany and Luxembourg.

Of course, one can speculate whether drinking wine or cooking with olive oil has a protective effect, but why focus on what people eat? The low mortality could as well be caused by any number of environmental, social or cultural factors typical of Mediterranean countries. The great difference in the number of heart attacks between the Mediterranean islands Crete and Corfu, for instance, cannot be explained by their blood cholesterol or their food because no measurable differences exist in these areas. Yet residents of Corfu have a five-fold higher risk of dying from CHD and suffer heart attacks 16 times more often than the inhabitants of Crete.[28]

Only by adding Japan and China to the data base were the authors of MONICA able to give some semblance of a correlation between blood cholesterol and risk of heart disease. But at least in Japan, other observations indicate that their low rate of coronary disease has nothing to do with their low cholesterol levels.

The Japanese paradox

The Japanese have low cholesterol levels and low rates of heart disease. This has been known for a long time and was confirmed by the Seven Countries study. Dr. Keys also found that Japanese immigrants to the mainland USA had high blood cholesterol and died almost as often from heart attacks as Americans did. The figures for Japanese immigrants to Hawaii lay somewhere in between.

Dr. Keys was convinced that the difference was caused by food, which in Japan is lean (at least it was when Keys performed his studies), while on Hawaii, and especially in the continental US, it is rich in animal fat.[29]

As usual, Keys had no other explanation. And he neglected to mention the fact that while coronary mortality increased after the Japanese had migrated to the US, stroke mortality decreased by the same amount and total mortality decreased much more.[30]

There is also an alternative explanation to the increased coronary mortality after migration from Japan to the US. As I mentioned earlier, calories from animal fat are usually expensive, and such food is therefore mostly consumed in rich countries, such as the Western, industrialized nations.

Calories from carbohydrates and vegetable oils are cheaper, and such food therefore predominates in poor countries with a low degree of industrialization and a low standard of living. When Ancel Keys gathered his data in the early 1960s, Japan belonged to this category. It was still poor, successfully recovering from war, not the rich nation, triumphant in industry, that we know today.

Immigrants from a poor country are exposed in their new, richer country to many other things besides high-fat food. A multitude of factors in the Western environment or lifestyle may adversely affect the heart and the blood vessels, such as less physical activity, more stress and more environmental and industrial pollutants. Furthermore, western doctors may also be more likely to use the diagnosis "heart attack" on the death certificate than Japanese doctors. In Japan, it is considered shameful to die of a heart attack but honorable to die from stroke.

In his doctoral thesis about coronary heart disease in Japanese immigrants, British physician Dr. Michael Marmot presents some interesting insights into the relationship be-

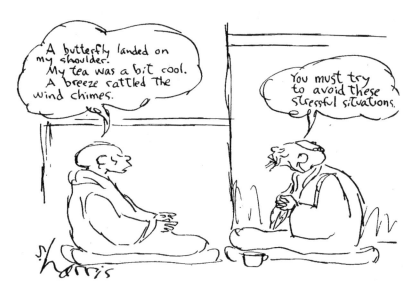

© 2000 by Sidney Harris

tween blood cholesterol levels and social factors, eating habits and lifestyle.[31] Dr. Marmot demonstrated that it was not the food that raised the cholesterol of the Japanese immigrants, nor high cholesterol values that increased their risk of coronary heart disease. He found that if they maintained their cultural traditions, they were protected against heart attacks, even though their cholesterol increased as much as in Japanese immigrants who adopted a Western lifestyle and who died from heart attacks almost as often as did native-born Americans. The most striking aspect of Dr. Marmot's findings was that *immigrants who became accustomed to the American way of life, but preferred lean Japanese food, had coronary disease twice as often as those who maintained Japanese traditions but preferred high-fat American food.*

Thus, according to Dr. Marmot's study, there is something in the Japanese lifestyle that protects against coronary heart disease, and it is not the food.

Dr. Marmot himself postulated protective factors in the traditional Japanese culture, which is still a major factor shaping life in present-day Japan. In particular, the Japanese place great emphasis on group cohesion, group achievement and social stability. Members of the stable Japanese society enjoy support from other members of their society and thus are protected from the emotional and social stress that Marmot believes to be an important cause of heart attacks. The Japanese traditions of togetherness contrast dramatically with the typical American emphasis on social and geographic mobility, individualism and striving ambition.

Ignoring embarrassing data

We do not know whether Dr. Marmot's explanation is correct. However, if his *findings* are correct, the diet-heart idea must be wrong. But Dr. Marmot's results, as well as many other embarrassing contradictory findings, have been ignored in official reviews.

In 1979, for instance, the American Health Foundation organized an international conference to determine "the optimal cholesterol level" with a view to adopting measures to lower cholesterol in countries where the conference participants thought it was too high. The written report from this conference[32] presented a meticulous account of Dr. Marmot's results, including detailed information about Japanese food, cholesterol levels and risk of heart disease. However, Marmot's message—and the epidemiological data on which it was founded—was ignored. The American Health Foundation report made no mention of the fact that the increased risk of coronary heart disease could not possibly be caused by the Japanese people's food or their blood cholesterol.

Let's look at a few more examples of researchers sweeping contradictory findings under the rug. A large review written in 1984 by Dr. William Kannel, head of the Framingham project, and his colleagues, stated that "there is a strong association between population means of total cholesterol and CHD incidence."[33] ("Total cholesterol" simply means "cholesterol." The term "total cholesterol" is used in texts where subfractions such as LDL- and HDL-cholesterol are also mentioned.)

The reference Dr. Kannel gives for this statement is the Seven Countries study. He doesn't mention the fact that Keys' data show no significant correlation between blood cholesterol and coronary disease.

The largest official review on heart disease, *Diet and Health*, written in 1989, comes from the prestigious National Research Council. The report concludes as follows: "Epidemiological findings among populations and for individuals within populations consistently indicate a strong, continuous, and positive relationship between TC [Total Cholesterol] levels and the prevalence and incidence of, as well as mortality from, atherosclerotic CHD."[34] But as I have demonstrated, this statement is far from the truth.

Typical of the inappropriate use of data to promote the

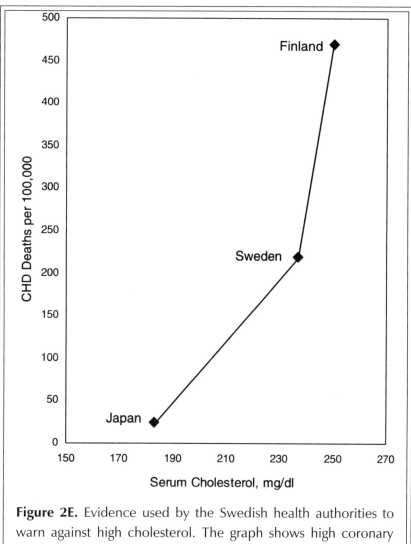

Figure 2E. Evidence used by the Swedish health authorities to warn against high cholesterol. The graph shows high coronary mortality in Finland, where blood cholesterol is high, and low coronary mortality in Japan, where blood cholesterol is low.

Source: Lars Wilhelmsen.

diet-heart idea is the graph shown in Figure 2E. It was prepared by Dr. Lars Wilhelmsen, one of the strongest supporters of the diet-heart idea in Sweden, and also one of the collaborators in the MONICA project. The graph illustrates the alleged association between blood cholesterol and CHD mortality in Japan, Sweden and Finland. Dr. Wilhelmsen's graph was often used previously by the official health authorities to warn Swedish doctors and the Swedish population about the dangers of high cholesterol.

The figure correctly shows that cholesterol is high in Finland, where heart attacks are common, and low in Japan, where heart attacks are rare, and that Sweden lies in between. At first glance, the graph seems convincing—the higher the cholesterol in the blood, the greater the risk of heart attack.

Now compare Dr. Wilhelmsen's graph with that of Figure 2D. Both figures are constructed in the same way, with blood cholesterol on the horizontal axis and coronary mortality on the vertical axis. But by leaving out most of the data points, Dr. Wilhelmsen gives us an incorrect impression of a strong correlation.

Of course, Dr. Wilhelmsen hasn't drawn the figure to deceive. Instead, wishful thinking combined with eagerness to educate the public has led him to oversimplify. But to do that, he has ignored all those irritating contradictory observations.

Many supporters of the diet-heart idea seem to have stopped thinking critically. Perhaps, as members of a worldwide alliance that includes many distinguished researchers, they have become overconfident, too willing to assume that an idea must surely be valid if great numbers of people endorse it. But if they were familiar with the way science has progressed through the centuries, they would know that the truth cannot be suppressed by the majority or decreed by consensus.

Another myth: " Good" and "bad" cholesterol

Cholesterol is a peculiar molecule. It is often called a lipid or a fat, but the chemical term for a molecule such as cholesterol is alcohol, although it doesn't behave like alcohol. Its numerous carbon and hydrogen atoms are put together in an intricate three-dimensional network, impossible to dissolve in water. All living creatures use this indissolubility cleverly, incorporating cholesterol into their cell walls to make cells waterproof, a mechanism vital for proper function. Cholesterol in the cell walls of living creatures leaves regulation of the internal cellular environment relatively undisturbed by chemical changes in the surrounding milieu. The fact that cells are waterproof is especially critical for normal functioning of nerves and nerve cells. Thus, the highest concentration of cholesterol in the body is found in the brain and other parts of the nervous system.

Because cholesterol is insoluble, it circulates in the blood inside spherical particles composed of fats (lipids) and proteins, the so-called lipoproteins. Lipoproteins are easily dissolved in water because their outside is composed mainly of water-soluble proteins. The inside is composed of lipids, with room for water-insoluble molecules like cholesterol. Like submarines, lipoproteins carry cholesterol through the blood from one place in the body to another.

These submarines, or lipoproteins, are categorized according to their density. The best known are HDL (High Density Lipoprotein) and LDL (Low Density Lipoprotein).

The main task of HDL is to carry cholesterol from the peripheral tissues, including the artery walls, to the liver. Here it is excreted with the bile or used for other purposes.

The LDL submarines mainly transport cholesterol in the opposite direction. They carry it from the liver, where most of our body's cholesterol is produced, to the peripheral tissues, including the blood vessel walls. When cells need extra cholesterol, they call for the LDL submarines, which then deliver cholesterol into the interior of the cells.

Between 60 and 80 percent of the cholesterol in the blood is transported by LDL and is called "bad" cholesterol. Only 15-20 percent is transported by HDL and is called "good" cholesterol. An additional small part of the circulating cholesterol is transported by other types of lipoproteins.

You may ask why a natural substance in our blood, with important biological functions, is called "bad" when it is transported from the liver to the peripheral tissues by LDL but "good" when it is transported in the other direction by HDL. The reason is that a number of follow-up studies have shown that a lower-than-normal level of HDL-cholesterol and a higher-than-normal level of LDL-cholesterol are associated with a greater risk of having a heart attack; and, conversely, that a higher-than-normal level of HDL-cholesterol and a lower-than-normal level of LDL-cholesterol are associated with a smaller risk. Or, said in another way, a low HDL/LDL ratio is a risk factor for coronary heart disease.

By now you know that a risk factor is not necessarily the same as the cause, and that something may provoke a heart attack and at the same time lower the HDL/LDL ratio. Let's have a look at some factors known to influence this ratio.

The cholesterol ratio caper

As mentioned above, people who reduce their body weight also reduce their cholesterol. A review of 70 studies, performed by Drs. A. M. Dattilo and P. M. Kris-Etherton at the Department of Foods and Nutrition, University of Georgia, showed that, on average, weight reduction lowers cholesterol by about 10 percent, depending on the amount of weight lost.[23] Interestingly, it is only cholesterol transported by LDL that goes down during weight loss; the small part transported by HDL goes up. In other words, weight reduction increases the ratio between HDL and LDL cholesterol.

Diet-heart supporters say that an increased HDL/LDL ratio is favorable; cholesterol is changed from "bad" to "good." But is it the ratio or the weight reduction that is favorable? When we become fat, other harmful things occur. One is that our cells become less sensitive to insulin, so much so that some of us even develop diabetes. And people with diabetes are much more likely to have a heart attack than people without diabetes because atherosclerosis and other vascular damage may occur early in diabetics, even in those with normal cholesterol. Also, overweight is often due to inactivity, and inactivity predisposes to heart disease. (See below.) In other words, overweight may increase the risk of a heart attack by mechanisms other than an abnormal HDL/LDL ratio, while at the same time overweight lowers the HDL/LDL ratio.

You may also recall that smoking increases cholesterol a little. Again, it is LDL-cholesterol that increases, while HDL-cholesterol goes down, resulting in an unfavorable HDL/LDL ratio.[22] What is certainly unfavorable is chronic exposure to the fumes from burning paper and tobacco leaves. In Chapter 7, I shall discuss how such fumes may endanger the blood vessels, but it should already be obvious that instead of considering a low HDL/LDL ratio as bad, we should consider the possibility that smoking in and of itself is bad. Smoking may provoke a heart attack and, at the same time, lower the HDL/LDL ratio.

Exercise decreases the so-called bad LDL-cholesterol and increases the so-called good HDL-cholesterol.[35] In fact, in well-trained individuals the good HDL is increased considerably. In a comparison between distance runners and sedentary individuals, Dr. Paul D. Thompson and his team from Providence, Rhode Island found that athletes had, on average, a 41 percent higher HDL-cholesterol level.[36] Most population studies have shown that physical exercise is associated with a lower risk of heart attack and a sedentary life with a higher risk. A well-trained heart is better guarded against obstruction of the coronary vessels than a heart always working at low speed simply because the vascular channels in the well-trained heart are broader— remember the wide coronary vessels of the Masai in Kenya who ran all day long after their cattle. A sedentary life may predispose people to a heart attack and, at the same time, lower the HDL/LDL ratio.

A low ratio is also associated with high blood pressure.[24]

Most often, hypertension is created by a sympathetic nervous system that is stimulated by too much adrenaline, particularly when an individual is under a lot of stress. Hypertension may therefore provoke a heart attack—for instance, by an adrenaline-induced spasm of the coronary arteries—and, at the same time, lower the HDL/LDL ratio.

Univariate and multivariate

As you can see, it is not easy to know what is bad. Is it bad to be fat, to smoke, to be inactive, to have high blood pressure or to be under stress? Or is it bad to have a lot of so-called bad cholesterol? Or both? Is it good to be slim, to stop smoking, to exercise, to have normal blood pressure or to be emotionally calm? Or is it good to have a lot of so-called good cholesterol? Or both?

Thus, the risk of having a heart attack is greater than normal for people with high LDL-cholesterol, but so is the risk for fat, sedentary, smoking, hypertensive and mentally stressed individuals. And since such individuals usually have elevated levels of LDL-cholesterol, it is, of course, impossible to know whether the increased risk is due to the previously mentioned risk factors, or to risk factors we have not yet discovered, or to the high LDL-cholesterol alone. A calculation of the risk of high LDL-cholesterol that does not consider other risk factors is called a univariate analysis and is, of course, meaningless.

To prove that high LDL-cholesterol is an independent risk factor, we should ask whether fat, sedentary, smoking, hypertensive and mentally stressed individuals with high LDL-cholesterol are at greater risk for coronary disease than fat, sedentary, smoking, hypertensive and mentally stressed individuals with low or normal LDL-cholesterol.

Using complicated statistical formulas, it is possible to do such comparisons in a population of individuals with varying degrees of risk factors and varying levels of LDL-cholesterol, a so-called multivariate analysis. If a multivariate analysis of the prognostic influence of LDL-cholesterol also takes body weight into consideration, it is said to be adjusted for body weight.

A major problem with such calculations is that we know about a great number of risk factors, and the more risk factors that are adjusted for, the less reliable the result will be. Another problem is that the data generated by these and other complicated statistical methods are almost impossible for most readers—including most doctors—to comprehend. For many years researchers in this area have not presented primary data, simple means or simple correlations. Instead, their papers have been salted with meaningless ratios, relative risks and p-values, not to mention obscure concepts such as the standardized logistic regression coefficient or the pooled hazard rate ratio. Instead of being an aid to science, statistics are used to impress the reader and cover up the fact that the scientific findings are trivial and without practical importance. Nevertheless, let's have a look at some of the studies.

"Good" cholesterol

Publications almost beyond counting have studied the prognostic value of "good" HDL-cholesterol. The trouble is that it is hard to find any prognostic value. If HDL-cholesterol had a heart-protecting effect of real importance, it would not be necessary to use taxpayer money for expensive studies to demonstrate the effect over and over again. To be brief, we'll look at only a few of the largest studies.

In 1986 Dr. Stuart Pocock and his team from London and Birmingham, England, published a report concerning more than 7000 middle-aged men in 24 British towns.[37] The men had been followed for about four years after a detailed analysis of their blood. During this period, 193 of the men had a heart attack. As in most previous studies, these men had lower than average HDL-cholesterol at the beginning of the study than the men who did not have a heart attack. The mean difference between those who had a heart attack and the other men was about 6 percent. This difference was small, of course, but thanks to the large number of individuals studied, it was statistically significant.

But this was a univariate analysis and, as mentioned, the difference could therefore be explained in many ways. A multivariate analysis adjusted for age, blood pressure, body weight, cigarette smoking and non-HDL-cholesterol reduced the difference to an insignificant 2 percent. This means that those who had suffered a heart attack had a lower HDL-cholesterol mainly because they were older, fatter, had higher blood pressure and smoked more than those who had not had a heart attack.

The British scientists compared their findings with those of six other studies. In five of them the differences were just as small. Only one study found a considerable difference, but it included only 39 individuals and thus was highly susceptible to bias. Dr. Pocock and his colleagues concluded that low HDL-cholesterol is not a major risk factor for coronary heart disease.

Their results were challenged in 1989 by nine American scientists headed by Dr. David Gordon at the National Heart, Lung and Blood Institute. They analyzed the predictive value of HDL-cholesterol in four large American studies, including a total of more than 15,000 men and women.[38] They thought that the British scientists had used an incorrect method to obtain their figures. According to Dr. Gordon and his team, HDL-cholesterol could be shown to be a much better predictor for heart disease if another method of statistical analysis were used.

What Dr. Gordon and his team discovered was that changing the method of statistical analysis did *not* result in more comfortable conclusions. In one of the four studies that Dr. Gordon and his colleagues analyzed, the number of fatal heart attacks was identical in the first and second HDL tertile.

(Individuals were assigned to three groups, or tertiles, according to the level of their HDL-cholesterol.) In another of the studies, the number of fatal cases was identical in the second and the third tertile, and in one study more deaths were seen in the third tertile (those who had the largest amount of the "good" cholesterol) than in the second tertile. And these figures were the unadjusted ones.

After adjustment for age, cigarette smoking, blood pressure, body weight and LDL-cholesterol, the differences were even smaller. In three of the four studies, the differences lost statistical significance. And remember that the figures were not adjusted for physical activity or mental stress, not to mention risk factors we have not yet discovered.

Dr. Pocock and his colleagues returned to the subject with a new analysis later the same year, using the same method that Dr. Gordon and his colleagues had used. At that time the participants in the study had been followed for more than seven years, and a total of 443 heart attacks had occurred.[39]

This time a difference was noted between the HDL-cholesterol of the heart patients and the others. The difference was small but statistically significant, even after adjustment for the five major risk factors. However, the largest difference was noted for total cholesterol. The authors therefore concluded that a determination of HDL-cholesterol may be of marginal additional value in screening and in intervention programs for risk of coronary heart disease. They could also have added that as they did not adjust for *all* risk factors, the difference could as well have been due to the fact that the heart attack patients were more stressed or less physically active than the others.

And even if the difference had remained after adjustment of all the known risk factors, the crucial question is whether HDL-cholesterol has any importance whatsoever. I have shown that there is little or no evidence that blood cholesterol plays any role at all in coronary heart disease. If total cholesterol—

Table 2A. Mean HDL-cholesterol in three Finnish areas and coronary mortality 24 years later.

	Initial HDL-Cholesterol mg/dl	CHD Deaths per 1000 men (standardized)
Helsinki	44.8	81
West Finland	43.2	105
North Karelia	47.6	183

After Keys.[40]

a better predictor than HDL-cholesterol—is unimportant, how could HDL-cholesterol be important?

I am tempted to discuss the many other studies that did not find HDL-cholesterol to be a good predictor, but to avoid boring you, I shall mention only the 24-year follow-up of the Finnish group in the Seven Countries study, because this is one of the longest follow-up studies of HDL-cholesterol.[40] Researchers followed a total of 518 healthy men from three areas in Finland. Table 2A gives the number of fatal heart attacks and the starting average HDL-cholesterol in each area.

If HDL-cholesterol were good for the heart, the smallest number of men should have died from heart attacks in North Karelia, where HDL-cholesterol was the highest. Instead, the number was more than twice as large as in Helsinki, where HDL-cholesterol was the lowest.

In their paper, Dr. Keys and his coauthors mentioned two equally large and long-lasting studies that also found lower HDL-cholesterol in the healthy survivors than in those who had died from coronary disease. But in the summary of the paper they wrote the following: "These 24-year findings are not necessarily in conflict with reports in the literature on an inverse relationship between coronary heart disease incidence and HDL-cholesterol."

It is fortunate that low HDL-cholesterol itself does not increase the risk of a heart attack, because the "prudent" diet has a surprising effect on the HDL-cholesterol level. A French study by Dr. Frédéric Fumeron and his colleagues in Paris and Lille investigated the effect of two different diets on 36 healthy individuals. One diet contained 70 grams of butter, the other 70 grams of sunflower margarine; otherwise the diets were similar. Each individual ate both diets for three weeks; half of them started with the butter diet, half with the "prudent" margarine diet.[41]

As in many previous studies, analysis of the blood lipids before and after each period showed that the "prudent" diet lowered blood cholesterol. But it also lowered the "good" HDL-cholesterol, especially two of its subfractions called HDL-2 and LpA-I. Other studies have shown that these subfractions are especially "good." The authors also reviewed seven other studies with similar results.

"Bad" cholesterol

"LDL has the strongest and most consistent relationship to individual and population risk of CHD, and LDL-cholesterol is centrally and causally important in the pathogenetic chain leading to atherosclerosis and CHD." Thus wrote the authors of the large US government review *Diet and Health*.[34]

A scientific review is, like this book, an analysis of what has been done and what has been written about a certain subject. Such reviews usually do not present observations or experiments performed by the authors themselves. Reviews help researchers by sparing them the tedious work of seeking the primary observations in the library or in the electronic data bases. Furthermore, scientific reviews allow researchers to refer to a few reviews instead of a large number of original works. But, of course, those who refer to reviews must be sure that they are complete and correct and that they give balanced views and accurate conclusions.

Reviews by distinguished scientific bodies are supposed to meet such standards. Therefore, you are probably wondering how the authors of *Diet and Health* reached their conclusion about LDL-cholesterol. I wondered, too, when I started to untangle the HDL-LDL issue, because extensive reading had not yet given me the answer.

The fact is that very few analyses of LDL-cholesterol have been published. For example, in the hundreds of reports from the Framingham study, very little is mentioned about LDL-cholesterol. This is odd because all participants had this cholesterol fraction measured at the start and again later in the study.

Diet and Health is the official, most authoritative and supposedly most reliable review from the National Research Council in Washington, DC. I was confident that its highly qualified authors would have the answer. What was their evidence? Upon which observations or experiments did they base their statements about the dangers of LDL-cholesterol?

Diet and Health cites four publications. First, in 1973 Dr. Jack Medalie and his team at the Tel Aviv University in Israel published a five-year follow-up study of 10,000 Israeli male government and municipal employees.[42] Among a large number of factors relevant to the study of coronary heart disease, they measured total and LDL-cholesterol. The participants were divided into three tertiles of similar size according to their total and LDL-cholesterol values. Those with the lowest values were placed in the first tertile, those with the highest values in the third. In Table 2B you can see the initial cholesterol values in each tertile and the number of heart attacks these men had after five years.

Table 2B shows, in accordance with many other studies, that more heart attacks occurred among those with the highest cholesterol levels. The differences were not impressive, how-

Table 2B. Numbers of heart attacks after five years (adjusted for age) according to initial level of total and LDL-cholesterol.

		TERTILE	
	First	**Second**	**Third**
Total Cholesterol mg/dl	77-189	190-219	220-500
Number of heart attacks per 1000 men	29	39	60
LDL-cholesterol mg/dl	40-149	150-189	190-460
Number of heart attacks per 1000 men	33	38	58

Data from Medalie.[42]

ever, considering that the figures were not adjusted for anything but age, which means that the third tertile simply may have included more stressed, overweight, inactive and smoking individuals than the first tertile.

Now to the most important point. According to *Diet and Health*, LDL-cholesterol has the strongest relationship to risk of coronary heart disease and should therefore be a better predictor than total cholesterol. As you can see, it was not. Instead, there was a larger difference in numbers of heart attacks between the first and third tertiles of total cholesterol

(29 and 60 heart attacks) than of LDL-cholesterol (33 and 58 heart attacks). In other words, the *Diet and Health* authors should not have cited the Israeli study as supporting the claim that elevated LDL-cholesterol is the most important predictor of heart disease, because in this study *total* cholesterol, not LDL-cholesterol, had the strongest relationship to risk of coronary disease.

The second paper cited in *Diet and Health* to support the idea about "dangerous" LDL-cholesterol was a 1977 report from the Framingham study.[43] But this study concerned mainly HDL-cholesterol. The only information about LDL-cholesterol that was given to support their conclusions was logistic regression coefficients—a statistical concept unknown to most doctors. One of the study's conclusions was that "LDL-cholesterol. . . is a marginal risk factor for people of these age groups" (men and women above 50 years). Some of the coefficients were indeed low. For women above the age of 70 it was negative, which means that women at that age ran a greater risk of having a heart attack if their LDL-cholesterol was low than if it was high. Thus, there was no support from the second reference either.

The third study cited[44] concerned only HDL-cholesterol. Once again, no support.

The fourth reference was to the National Cholesterol Education Program, which produced another large review without original data.[45] One of its conclusions was that "a large body of epidemiological evidence supports a direct relationship between the level of serum total and LDL-cholesterol and the rate of CHD."

"At last!" I thought. "The evidence I have been seeking!"

The "large body of evidence" turned out to be a mere three references.

One of the references was another large review[46] that made no mention of LDL-cholesterol.

Another one was a report from the Honolulu Heart study,[47]

which concluded that "both measures of LDL-cholesterol were related to CHD prevalence, but neither appeared to be superior to total cholesterol."

The third reference was yet another large review without original data, "Optimal resources for primary prevention of atherosclerotic disease,"[48] with Dr. Kannel as the first author. Almost nothing was written about LDL-cholesterol in Dr. Kannel's review except the following: "Longitudinal [longterm follow-up] studies within populations show a consistent rise in the risk of CHD in relation to serum total cholesterol and LDL-cholesterol at least until late middle-age."

Thus, Dr. Kannel's conclusion is more cautious than the conclusion as it appeared in *Diet and Health*, but even though Dr. Kannel chose his words more carefully, the evidence is weak. Kannel cites six studies as references. In two of them LDL-cholesterol was not analyzed or mentioned at all.[49] In two reports LDL-cholesterol was correlated only to the prevalence of heart disease, which means they were not longitudi-

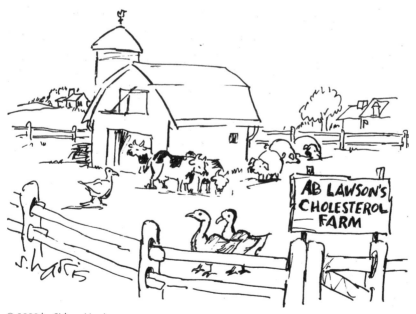

nal studies and thus they could not tell anything about the predictive value of LDL-cholesterol.[50] Another report dedicated two tables to the subject (Tables 8 and 9), which showed that the predictive power of LDL-cholesterol was statistically non-significant.[51] And in the final study, LDL-cholesterol was predictive for heart disease, but only for men between ages 35 and 49 and only for women between ages 40 and 44.[52]

In conclusion, the "large body of evidence" can be reduced to one single study, which showed a predictive value for LDL-cholesterol but only for a few age groups. The only valid conclusion, therefore, is that LDL-cholesterol is neither centrally nor causally important; it does not have the strongest and most consistent relationship to risk of CHD; and it lacks a direct relationship to the rate of CHD.

Endorsement of LDL-cholesterol as a risk factor is not the only erroneous conclusion promulgated by the National Cholesterol Education Program. In fact, this document is loaded with misquotations and even false statements.[53] The Program's endorsement of the use of drugs for CHD is also highly suspect. "The issue of whether lowering LDL-cholesterol levels by dietary and drug interventions can reduce the incidence of CHD has been addressed in more than a dozen randomized clinical trials," wrote the authors. This is a most misleading statement because at that time, in 1988, only four such trials had included an LDL-cholesterol analysis,[54] none of them succeeded in lowering heart disease mortality, and only one of them lowered nonfatal heart disease significantly.

Why LDL?

How was it that the idea of so-called "bad" cholesterol came to the fore? The National Cholesterol Education Program cites two main reasons. First was the discovery of a defective LDL-receptor in those with familial hypercholesterolemia and, in consequence, the extremely high level of LDL-cholesterol in the blood of individuals with this disease. The discoverers, Nobel prize winners Michael Brown and Joseph Goldstein, suggested that it was high LDL-cholesterol that caused the vascular changes seen in such individuals and, furthermore, that a similar mechanism was operating in the rest of us.[55] Second, feeding experiments in animals raised the animals' LDL-cholesterol and produced vascular changes that experimenters have labeled "atherosclerosis." (More about animal experiments in Chapter 5.)

But these arguments are weak. If LDL-cholesterol were the devil himself, LDL would clearly serve as a better predictor than total cholesterol, because the total cholesterol also includes the so-called "good" HDL-cholesterol. And experiments on animals are only suggestive and cannot prove anything about human diseases. Besides, as I shall discuss later, the vascular findings in laboratory animals do not look like human atherosclerosis at all, and it is impossible to induce a heart attack in animals by diet alone. Finally, findings pertaining to people with a rare genetic error in cholesterol metabolism are not necessarily valid for the rest of us.

Thus, the experimenters claim support from unsupportive epidemiological and clinical studies, and the epidemiologists and the clinicians claim support from inconclusive experimental evidence. The victim of this miscarriage of justice is an innocent and useful molecular construction in our blood, producers and manufacturers of animal fat all over the world, and millions of healthy people who are frightened and badgered into eating a tedious and flavorless diet that is said to lower their "bad" cholesterol.

The alleged influence of the diet on blood cholesterol is the subject of the next chapter.

TRIGLYCERIDES

Most of the fatty acids in the diet and in the blood are bound to a type of alcohol called glycerol. Usually each glycerol molecule is attached to three fatty acids, and this molecular complex is called a triglyceride, often shortened to TG. As with cholesterol, high TG levels in the blood have been found to be associated with an increased risk of CHD. Does that mean that we should lower the level of triglycerides in our blood to avoid CHD?

To answer this question satisfactorily demands careful reading and a long explanation. However, if you understand the fallacy of the cholesterol hypothesis, then it will be easy for you to understand that you do not need to bother about your triglycerides either, because even the most zealous proponents of pharmaceutical intervention admit that the evidence for high triglycerides causing atherosclerosis and cardiovascular disease is weak, much weaker than for high cholesterol. Thus, if it is weak or nonexistent for cholesterol, why bother about triglycerides?

The triglyceride level in the blood depends on many factors. Normally TGs go up after a meal. The more fats and carbohydrates you eat—and the more alcohol you drink—the higher your TG level becomes. Almost 12 hours must pass before the level returns to "normal." An analysis of triglycerides is therefore meaningless if the patient hasn't been fasting the previous 12 hours.

Furthermore, overweight people have higher levels of triglycerides in their blood than thin people, smokers have more than nonsmokers, diabetics have more than non-diabetics, people who lead a sedentary lifestyle have more than physically active people, and people under stress have more than people who are at ease. For instance, you could ask whether overweight, smoking, inactive and stressed diabetics with high triglycerides are more at risk than overweight, smoking, inactive and stressed diabetics with normal triglyceride levels.

In addition, analysis of triglycerides is highly inaccurate and the normal fasting levels are highly variable. If a blood analysis finds 200 mg per deciliter, the true TG level may be anything between 100 and 300. To get a more reliable measure of your normal TGs, it is therefore necessary to calculate the average of three measurements made at three different occasions, each time preceded by a 12-hour fast.

So, when researchers say that high triglycerides predict an increased risk for CHD, the question is whether this is caused by sedentary lifestyle, or smoking, or overweight, or mental stress, or diabetes, or a risk factor we don't know about yet; or whether it is caused by a high triglyceride level. And even if a 10-20 percent higher fasting value of TG is associated with an increased risk, it seems senseless to try to lower TG levels when TGs rise after each meal to levels that can be several hundred percent higher than the fasting state. All of us who eat three times a day and drink a glass of wine or whisky now and then simply have "too high" TG values in our blood most of the time.

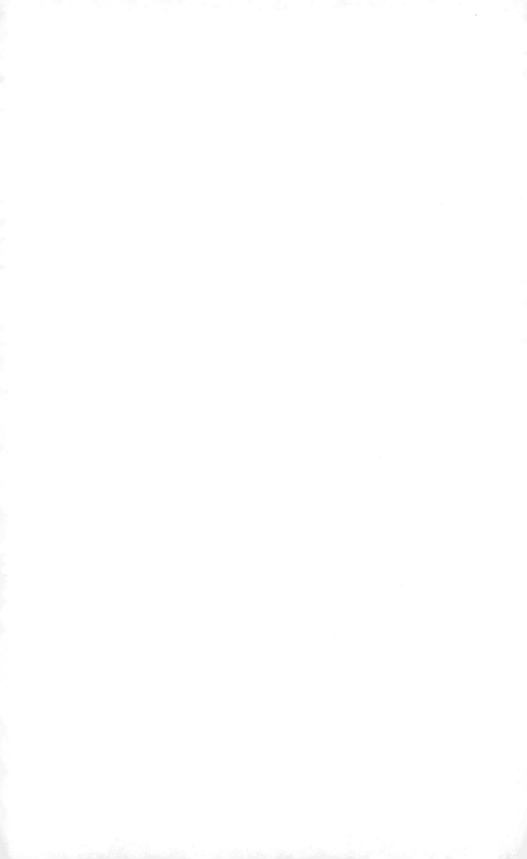

Myth 3

High-Fat Foods Raise Blood Cholesterol

Ye shall eat the fat of the land.
Genesis 45:18

Food and fat in various populations

Why do levels of cholesterol in the blood vary in different people? Because of their food! This is the answer from diet-heart proponent Ancel Keys, stated over and over again in his papers. No alternative explanations are ever mentioned; Dr. Keys' hand never trembles when he writes about the influence of diet on blood cholesterol.

One of his arguments is that the average blood cholesterol level is high in countries where people eat lots of high-fat food, especially foods high in animal fat, and low in countries where people eat little fat. And, asserts Keys, if an individual with low cholesterol moves to an area where people's cholesterol is high, then his cholesterol will also rise.

In 1958, Dr. Keys illustrated his idea with a diagram demonstrating the relationship between the amount of fat in the food and the cholesterol level of the blood in various populations.[1] (See Figure 3A.)

It is possible to draw a straight line through almost all the points that Keys selected, an amazing result considering the un-

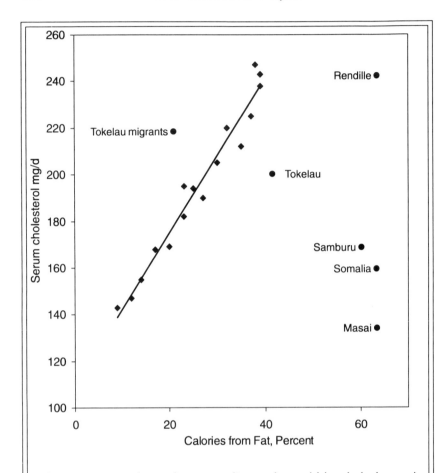

Figure 3A. Correlation between dietary fat and blood cholesterol in various populations. The squares represent populations selected by Ancel Keys. The circles represent some of the populations that Keys ignored. After Keys.[1]

certainties associated with the data behind the individual points. It is highly unusual to find such a strong correlation in medical or biological science because observations of living creatures are much more imprecise than observations in the fields of physics or chemistry.

Note also that the figure relates blood cholesterol to the total amount of dietary fat. In his Seven Countries study, published later, Dr. Keys claimed that the correlation was far better if cholesterol were related to the intake of animal fat only, rather than total fat. You may wonder how the correlation could be any better than the one Keys found in Figure 3A. The reason is that in the Seven Countries study, Keys found no correlation at all between total fat and heart mortality.

How come Dr. Keys found a strong correlation in the first study when in Seven Countries he found no correlation at all? Part of the answer is that in his first study, Dr. Keys followed his usual standard and left out population groups that didn't fit his theory.

Camels, cows and cholesterol

I have already discussed the discrepancies between the low blood cholesterol of the Masai and Samburu cattle herders and their rich, high-fat food. Why didn't Dr. Keys include these groups in his elegant diagram? Didn't he find it interesting that for long periods the Samburu drink over one gallon of milk each day? Milk from African Zebu cattle is much higher in fat than milk from modern Holstein cows, which means that the Samburu consume more than twice the amount of animal fat than the average milk-drinking American, and yet their cholesterol is much lower, about 170 mg/dl.[2]

Shepherds in Somalia consume almost nothing but milk from their camels. About a gallon and a half a day is normal, which amounts to at least one pound of butterfat, because camel's milk is much richer in fat than cow's milk. But although more than 60 percent of their energy consumption comes from animal fat, their mean cholesterol is only about 150 mg/dl, far lower than that of most Western people.[3]

Cholesterol and coconuts

Dr. Ian Prior and his team from Wellington, New Zealand, studied the population of the Tokelau Islands and the Pukapuka atolls,[4] where the main food is coconuts prepared in various ways.

Seafood and chicken are also on the menu. Coconuts contain great amounts of coconut oil. Unlike most other types of vegetable fat, coconut is high in saturated fatty acids. In fact, coconut oil is more saturated than animal fat.

On the Tokelau Islands the amount of saturated fat was almost twice that of Pukapuka and even higher than in the US, while consumption of polyunsaturated oils was low on all islands.

The scientists confirmed that the Polynesians really ate this great amount of saturated fatty acids by analyzing the fat beneath their skin. They removed a little of this fat with a syringe and found that its content of saturated fatty acids was twice that of Western people. Also, the chickens these Pacific islanders ate had a high content of saturated fatty acids in their fat, probably because they also consumed a considerable amount of coconut.

The cholesterol of the Tokelauans was higher than that of the Pukapuka inhabitants, as expected according to the diet-heart idea, but it was at least 20 percent lower than it should have been if Dr. Keys' calculations were correct.

But the most interesting part of this study became apparent later. In 1966, a tornado pulled up a great number of coconut trees on the islands. The atolls could no longer feed their inhabitants, and one thousand Tokelauans migrated to New Zealand. In New Zealand their diet changed markedly; the number of calories from saturated fat was cut in half while the intake of polyunsaturated fat increased a small amount.[5]

Here was the perfect opportunity to prove the diet-heart hypothesis, but the results of this so-called "favorable" change in diet did not live up to expectations. Instead of going down as expected, the cholesterol of the Tokelauans increased by about 10 percent, as seen in Table 3A.

Thus, something in the environment or life-style in New Zealand had such a great impact on the Tokelauans that their cholesterol levels increased, although their consumption of saturated fat was reduced by half.

Table 3A. Fat content of the food of Tokelau inhabitants and Tokelau immigrants in New Zealand, and their blood cholesterol levels.

	Tokelau	New Zealand
Proportion energy (%) from		
saturated fat	45	21
polyunsaturated fat	3	4
Blood cholesterol (mg/dl)		
men, 45-54 years	195	219
women, 45-54 years	213	225

Data from Stanhope, Sampson and Prior.[5]

Experiments and reality

Another of Dr. Keys' arguments derives from the results of laboratory experiments to lower cholesterol by diet. The experiments are summarized as follows: If energy is supplied mainly by saturated fatty acids, the type of fats found mainly in animal fat and in coconut butter, blood cholesterol goes up a little; if energy is supplied mainly by polyunsaturated fatty acids, the type of fats found mostly in vegetable oils and seafood, blood cholesterol goes down a little.

Oddly, cholesterol in the diet has only a marginal influence on the cholesterol in the blood. The explanation is that we regulate our own production of cholesterol according to our needs. When we eat large amounts of cholesterol, our body's production goes down; when we eat small amounts, it goes up.

The fact that a certain type of diet may change blood cholesterol levels has been demonstrated by the cholesterol-lowering trials. An extreme diet may lower the level by about 10 percent; a more palatable diet only a few percent.[6] We'll discuss this further in Chapter 6.

Now to one of the cholesterol paradoxes. Although it is possible to change blood cholesterol a little by diet in laboratory experiments and clinical trials, it is impossible to find any relationship between the makeup of the diet and the blood cholesterol of individuals who are not participating in a medical experiment. In other words, individuals who live as usual and eat their food without listening to doctors or dieticians show no connection between what they eat and the level of their blood cholesterol.

If the diet-heart idea were correct, individuals who eat large amounts of animal fat would have higher cholesterol levels than those who eat small amounts, and individuals who eat small amounts of vegetable oils would have higher cholesterol levels than those who eat large amounts. If this is not the case, then there is no reason to meddle with people's diets. (And even if it were true, there is still no reason for dietary intervention because, as seen from the previous chapter, high cholesterol is not the real cause of coronary heart disease.)

Counting money and counting food

Even in the early 1950s, the Framingham study included dietary analyses. Almost one thousand individuals were questioned in detail about their eating habits, but the researchers found no connection between the composition of the food and blood cholesterol levels. Drs. William Kannel and Tavia Gordon, authors of the report, wrote the following summary: "These findings suggest a cautionary note with respect to hypotheses relating diet to serum cholesterol levels. There is a considerable range of serum cholesterol levels within the Framingham Study Group. Something explains this inter-individual variation, but *it is not the diet.*"

For unknown reasons, their results were never published. The manuscript is still lying in a basement in Washington, DC.[7]

In a small American town called Tecumseh, in the state of Michigan, a similar study was performed by a team of researchers from the University of Michigan headed by Dr. Allen Nichols.

Experienced dieticians questioned more than two thousand individuals in great detail about what they had eaten during a 24-hour period. The dieticians also asked about the ingredients in the food, analyzed the recipes of home-cooked dishes and expended considerable effort to find out what kind of fat was used in the kitchen. Calculations were then performed using an elaborate list that provided the composition of almost 3000 American food items. Finally, the participants were divided into three groups—a high, a middle and a low-level group, according to their blood cholesterol.

No difference was found between the amounts of any food item in the three groups. Of special interest was the fact that the low-cholesterol group ate just as much saturated fat as did the high-cholesterol group.[8]

These studies concerned adults, but no association has been found in children either. At the famous Mayo Clinic in Rochester, Minnesota, for instance, Dr. William Weidman and his team analyzed the diet of about one hundred school children. Great differences were found in the amount of various food items eaten by these children, and also great differences in their blood cholesterol values, but there wasn't the slightest connection between the two. The children who ate lots of animal fat had just as much or just as little cholesterol in their blood as the children who ate very little animal fat.[9] A similar investigation of 185 children in New Orleans, the Bogalusa Heart study, gave the same result.[10]

Even when no pains are spared to investigate the diet of individuals and groups, the information gathered is, of course, uncertain. Who can recall everything that he has eaten within the past twenty-four hours? And the diet of one 24-hour period may not be representative of the usual diet. A better result can be achieved by studying the diet over several days, preferably during various seasons of the year. In London, professor Jeremy Morris and his team used this method and asked 99 middle-aged male bank staff members to weigh and record what they ate over two weeks.[11]

Have you ever bargained in a bank? Maybe you will succeed in the director's office, but certainly not at the teller's counter. If anyone is scrupulous with nickels and dimes, it is the person at the bank, sitting behind the glass.

Ninety-nine of these honorable men were asked to sit at home with a letter balance and weigh every morsel they ate for a whole week. But again, this meticulous method revealed no connection between the food they ate and their blood cholesterol levels.

To be certain, 76 of the bank men repeated the procedure for another week at another time of the year: once again, no connection between diet and blood cholesterol levels was found.

To be absolutely certain, the researchers selected those whose records were especially detailed and accurate. Once more, no connection was found.

Another look at Finland

Finnish people have, on average, the highest cholesterol values in the world. According to the diet-heart idea's proponents, this is due to high-fat Finnish food. The answer is not that simple, however. This was demonstrated by Dr. Rolf Kroneld and his team at the University of Turku.[12] They studied all inhabitants of the village of Iniö near Turku, and twice as many randomly selected individuals of the same age and sex in North Karelia and in southwest Finland.

Apparently a health campaign was already underway in Iniö as the consumption of margarine was twice as great and the consumption of butter only half of what it was in the other Finnish districts. Furthermore, the people of Iniö preferred skimmed over whole milk while the residents of other districts did not. But the highest cholesterol values were found in Iniö.

The average value for male Iniö inhabitants was 283 mg/dl compared to 239 and 243 in the other two districts. For women, the difference was even greater.

Threshold on trial

Is it really wise to meddle with people's dietary habits if their food has no influence on their cholesterol? And how do those who believe that high-fat food is dangerous explain all these negative results?

Most often they argue that information about dietary habits is inaccurate—and it is. But this objection is not applied consistently. It is never raised against the studies mentioned in Chapter 1, those that claimed a connection between fat intake and heart mortality in various countries, although the uncertainty in those studies was much higher. The researchers did not determine dietary information by any questionnaires or surveys at all, but instead on estimates of the average intake of fat based on the highly uncertain assumption that people eat what is available. Such soft evidence should be treated with the utmost caution, but diet-heart supporters refuse to do more than applaud investigations that support their theories.

But even information gathered through direct questioning is inaccurate. A crude relationship should appear if a sufficiently large number of individuals are meticulously questioned. If not, the influence of the diet, if any, must be so weak that it cannot possibly have any importance.

Diet-heart supporters also argue that most people in Western communities already eat great amounts of fat and cholesterol. This argument declares that we have already crossed a threshold of too much animal fat in the diet so that more fat does not make any impact on our blood cholesterol.

The argument is in conflict with the studies I have mentioned above. Dr. Nichols and his team,[8] for instance, declared: "The distribution of daily intake of total fat, saturated fat, and cholesterol by the individuals in this study was quite broad." And indeed it was. For about 15 percent of the men, less than 12.8 percent of calories came from animal fat, and for about 15 percent of the men, more than 20 percent of the calories came from animal fat.

Consider now that it is the goal of the National Cholesterol Education Program to lower the intake of animal fat of all Americans to about 10 percent of their caloric intake. Almost 15 percent of the participants in the Tecumseh study already ate amounts of animal fat that low, and yet it was impossible to see a difference between the blood cholesterol of those who ate small amounts of animal fat and those who ate much more. Does it make sense to recommend this drastic reduction of animal fat if the cholesterol level of the ascetic is just as high as that of the epicure?

The Mayo Clinic study also revealed a wide range of fat intake. The lowest intake of animal fat was 15 grams per day (less than 10 percent of the caloric intake); the highest was 60 grams per day. In the Bogalusa study, the range was still broader. The lowest intake of *all* fats was 17 grams per day, the highest 325 grams per day. (No information about the relative proportion of animal fat to vegetable oil was given.)

In Jerusalem, a team of researchers led by Dr. Harold Kahn studied the diet and blood cholesterol of ten thousand male Israeli civil servants. The dietary habits varied considerably between people from Israel, Eastern Europe, Central Europe, Southern Europe, Asia and Africa. The intake of animal fat varied from 10 grams up to 200 grams daily, and there were also considerable differences between their cholesterol values.[13]

If the intake of animal fat were of major importance for the cholesterol levels in the blood, then it should be possible to find some kind of relationship from a study of so many individuals with such great variations in blood cholesterol and dietary habits. But there was no relation in this Israeli study either. Extremely low cholesterol values were seen both in those who ate small amounts of animal fat and in those who ate the most animal fat, and high cholesterol values were seen at all levels of animal-fat consumption.

The scientists from Israel also studied the value of various ways of dietary questioning. Many studies have recorded the diet during only one 24-hour period. Even if this information were accurate, it may not be representative of the diet for the rest of the year, far less for a whole lifetime. The Israeli scientists found that the best information came from surveys conducted over several days and during different seasons of the year, the method used in the study of the bank tellers. Using this expensive and time-consuming method in a smaller study of 62 individuals, researchers could not find any correlation either; the correlation coefficient between animal-fat intake and blood cholesterol was zero point zero. [14]

Vegetarians usually have lower cholesterol levels than other people, and they eat little animal fat. But vegetarians differ from the rest of the human population in more than their diet. They are usually more interested in their health, they usually smoke less, they are usually thinner and they usually exercise more often than other people. Whether it is their diet or their other living habits, or perhaps something else that lowers their blood cholesterol, is unknown.

There is a simple explanation for the fact that blood cholesterol is influenced by diet in laboratory experiments and clinical trials but not in people who live without the interference of scientists and dieticians: Blood cholesterol is controlled by more powerful factors than the diet. If these factors are kept reasonably constant in a laboratory experiment or a clinical trial, it is possible to see the influence of the diet alone.

The question, however, is whether a reduction of blood cholesterol by diet is permanent. As mentioned above, the body tends to keep its blood cholesterol at a fairly constant level. The dietary experiments mentioned above went on for a few months at most. The cholesterol control mechanisms of the human body probably need more time to adapt to fat intake levels that differ from the norm. Over millions of years, mammals, including *homo sapiens* (our kind of men), have developed effective mechanisms to maintain homeostasis, that is, to counteract unfavorable changes in all the various constituents of the blood. Salt and water, for instance, are effectively regulated to remain within narrow limits because even small deviations may have a strong influence on the functions of the body. Extreme variations of other substances, such as proteins and fats, have no serious consequences in the short run; the adaptation is thus slow. But in due time, these deviations may also be counteracted; this has been demonstrated by the Masai, Samburu, Somalian shepherds and many others.

Food and blood cholesterol

You may ask why I have written so much about fats. After all, it is blood cholesterol levels that matter, not the level of fats in the blood, and the most important thing should be how much cholesterol we eat, not how much fat. If we eat lots of cholesterol, doesn't our blood cholesterol increase? It is not that simple.

Have you limited your daily consumption of eggs, the richest source of cholesterol in our food? Do you search the shelves of the grocery store to find items that are cholesterol-free? If so, the following statement will either make you angry or allow you to breathe a sigh of relief: The cholesterol in your food has little or no influence at all on the cholesterol in your blood.

Even the most zealous proponents of the diet-heart idea know this very well, but publicly they keep silent, because how on earth can you promote the idea that high blood cholesterol is a threat while allowing people to eat as much cholesterol as they like? The truth is that cholesterol in your food can't influence your blood cholesterol by more than a few percent.

Numerous studies have shown that in people who eat a normal Western diet, the effect on blood cholesterol of eating two or three extra eggs per day over a long period of time can hardly be measured.[15]

Another way of studying the effect of dietary cholesterol is by asking many people about their usual diet and comparing their answers with their blood cholesterol. Some of the dietary studies mentioned above, for instance the Tecumseh study, [8] the study from the Mayo Clinic[9] and Professor Morris' study of bank tellers,[11] also included an analysis of how much cholesterol the participants ate each day. None of them found any association between the amount of cholesterol in the diet and the amount of cholesterol in the blood; in fact, in two of these studies,[8,9] those who ate the smallest amount of cholesterol had the highest levels of blood cholesterol. The differences were small, however, and did not reach what we call statistical significance.

To find out how egg consumption influenced my own blood cholesterol, I once used myself as a human guinea pig without asking the ethics committee at any university. Before and during the experiment I analyzed my cholesterol. My usual egg consumption is one or two eggs per day, and my cholesterol value at the start of the experiment was 278 mg/dl, very close to a determination of blood cholesterol made ten years earlier. The results are shown in Table 3B.

Table 3B. Egg consumption and cholesterol values in one skeptical Swedish doctor.

Day	Number of Eggs Consumed	Blood Cholesterol (mg/dl)
0	1	278
1	4	--
2	6	--
3	8	266
4	8	264
5	8	264
6	8	257
7	8	274
8	8	246

Of course, one should be careful about drawing conclusions from an experiment on a single individual. However, it is not forbidden to speculate a little; after all, eight eggs a day represent a substantial amount of cholesterol.

The data from my daring experiment show that instead of going up, my cholesterol went down a little, even though I was eating two or three times more cholesterol than my body normally produces itself. Why didn't my cholesterol go up?

Most probably, no change took place at all. Blood cholesterol measurement can never be as exact as measurements of your weight or height. If you take a large blood sample, divide it between nine test tubes and analyze the cholesterol concentration of each tube, you will probably get nine different values. The difference between the lowest and the highest of them can be as great as 15 percent or more, although the true concentration is, of course, identical in all nine samples. Normal day-to-day cholesterol variations make it even more difficult to get an accurate measurement. The small decline in my cholesterol could simply have been due to imprecise measurements.

What we do know is that when we eat large amounts of cholesterol, our cells slow down their own production of this vital substance. Part of the surplus in the blood is temporarily stored in the liver and part is excreted with the bile. In my case, this regulation was performed so efficiently that my blood cho-

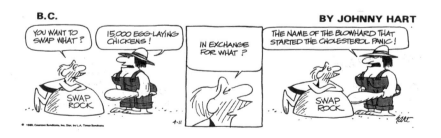

By permission of Johnny Hart and Creators Syndicate, Inc.

lesterol did not rise, in spite of a tenfold increase of my daily cholesterol intake. Perhaps my cholesterol would have finally gone up if I had continued longer with my experiment, but even if eggs are a good and nutritious food, who wants to eat eight eggs a day?

Proponents of the diet-heart idea would argue that I am what they call a "non-responder." According to this view, some members of the human race are able to maintain the same blood cholesterol levels even after having eaten large amounts of cholesterol. Maybe so, but in that case, most of mankind are non-responders. This can be deduced from a study performed by Dr. Martijn B. Katan and his group at the Department of Human Nutrition, Agricultural University in De Dreijen in the Netherlands.[16] The researchers began by giving 94 test individuals a low-cholesterol diet for two weeks, followed by a high-cholesterol diet (500 mg extra per day) for another two weeks. In 23 of the test individuals, called the hyper-responders, the cholesterol rose by 11 to 42 percent, whereas in 18, called the hypo-responders, the cholesterol change varied from a decrease (!) of 11 percent to an increase of 4 percent. These two groups, the hypo- and the hyper-responders, then participated in a second experiment, again with a high-cholesterol diet for two weeks. But this time the cholesterol changed very little, about 3 percent, and the change was about the same in each group. Thus, the experiment did not support the idea about hypo- and hyper-responders.

Surprised and disappointed with this unexpected result, the researchers decided to perform yet another experiment, this time with a total intake of almost one gram of cholesterol per day, and for three weeks instead of two. This time they got the results they wanted. Cholesterol increased in the hypo-responders by 9 percent and in the hyper-responders by 16 percent. But there was a lot of individual variation. As the authors wrote: "Quite a number of subjects who appeared hyper-responsive in one experiment proved to be hypo-responsive in another experiment."

To get a significant difference between the two groups, the

researchers resorted to the so-called one-tailed t-test, the less stringent parameter that is not accepted among scientists for use in research where the expected result can go in both directions—and here the result certainly went in both directions.

It is not particularly scientific either to continue an experiment until you get a result that suits your hypothesis, because sooner or later chance will produce a suitable result. And even if our cholesterol does rise a little after a meal rich in saturated fat and cholesterol, those who haven't skipped Chapter 2 know that high cholesterol is not necessarily dangerous to the heart.

But doesn't high cholesterol produce atherosclerosis?

This question is answered in the next chapter.

Myth 4

Cholesterol Blocks Arteries

Theorists almost always become too fond of their own ideas, often simply by living with them for so long. It is difficult to believe that one's cherished theory, which really works rather nicely in some respects, may become completely false.

Francis Crick, Nobel Prize Laureate
(together with James Watson,
for discovering the structure of DNA)

Cholesterol: Villain or innocent bystander?

Although scientists should do more questioning, in cholesterol research one statement never gets questioned because it is considered just as self-evident as the law of gravity. Even many opponents of the diet-heart idea neglect to question this statement. And what is this statement? It is that when cholesterol levels are high, it passes from the blood through the vessel walls, transforming arteries from smooth canals into rocky rapids.

Doctors and scientists may debate whether the cholesterol leaks in passively or is actively transported by the cells, but they are in general agreement about the importance of the cholesterol level in the blood; the higher it is, the faster the arteries become sclerotic.

As early as 1953, Ancel Keys wrote: "It is a fact that a major characteristic of the sclerotic artery is the presence of abnormal amounts of cholesterol in that artery." And he added: "This cholesterol is derived from the blood."[1]

No proofs and no arguments—not from Keys and not from his followers. The cholesterol comes from the blood, and that's the end to it. Scientists discuss how high the cholesterol level has to be for atherosclerosis to start, but they do not discuss whether the cholesterol level by itself has any importance. The role played by cholesterol in the process of atherosclerosis is no longer under discussion; it has been settled forever, or so we are led to believe.

Let's have a closer look at the facts.

Calcium and kidney stones

One finding that has convinced many scientists is the fact that when you inject radioactive cholesterol molecules into the blood, they show up at a later time in the atherosclerotic lesions. But calcium salts that end up as kidney stones were also circulating in the blood, once upon a time. It isn't possible, however, to prevent or eliminate kidney stones by lowering blood calcium levels, nor is it possible by lowering dietary calcium. And if we exclude a rare disease called hyperparathyroidism, calcium stones are certainly not due to high calcium levels in the blood because kidney stone patients do not have higher levels of calcium compared to those who are free of kidney stones.

Calcium salts in kidney stones originate from the blood, but we simply do not know why and how they become organized in the kidneys as stones. Any substance in a pathological structure in our body has at some time been transported by the blood. Its presence in the structure, be it a kidney stone or a sclerotic plaque or anything else, doesn't necessarily mean that the structure is produced by a high level of this substance in the blood. That high blood cholesterol doesn't produce atherosclerosis is also evident from many studies.

If cholesterol molecules circulating in the blood tend to settle in the arterial wall and produce atherosclerosis only because the blood contains more of them than normal, then people with high blood cholesterol should, on average, be more sclerotic than people with low blood cholesterol. This is pure logic. The protagonists also claim that this is the case. But, as we shall see, they are wrong.

False correlations

There are many ways for scientists to find a false correlation, and false correlations can mislead both scientists and their readers. Good, sound science is difficult; false answers are all too easy, even for the scientist who means well.

Let us start with a situation in which we have recorded the blood cholesterol and the degree of atherosclerosis in a large number of dead individuals. To see if blood cholesterol and degree of atherosclerosis are related, we draw a diagram where blood cholesterol is read on the horizontal axis and the degree of atherosclerosis on the vertical axis, as in Figure 4A. We may now obtain a false correlation if we have put together young and old individuals in our study, because in most studies old people on average have higher cholesterol and more atherosclerosis than young people do. Therefore, the young individuals with their somewhat lower cholesterol and their low degree of atherosclerosis will mainly be represented by the symbols in the lower left part of the diagram, and the old ones with their somewhat higher cholesterol and much more pronounced atherosclerosis will probably be represented by the symbols in the upper right. Thus, if we do not know the age of the individuals being studied, we might think that there is a correlation between blood cholesterol and atherosclerosis, when in fact it is a correlation between cholesterol and age and between atherosclerosis and age.

It is therefore necessary to study narrow age groups. For a scientifically valid answer, the question to ask is whether someone aged 60 who has high blood cholesterol is more sclerotic than another 60-year-old person whose blood cholesterol is low.

A false correlation may also appear if the study includes

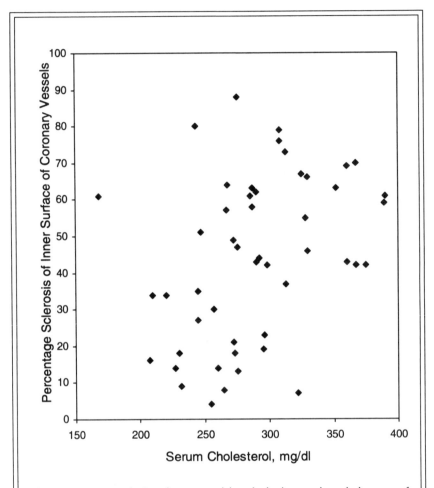

Figure 4A. Correlation between blood cholesterol and degree of coronary atherosclerosis in fifty middle-aged men. Beyond doubt, the highest cholesterol values (above 320) represent patients with familial hypercholesterolemia. Using all observations, there is a weak correlation (coefficient of correlation = 0.29). If the patients with presumed familial hypercholesterolemia are excluded, the correlation disappears.

Data from Solberg LA and others. In Schettler G, Goto Y, Hata Y, Klose G (ed.), *International Symposium of IV*. pages 98-102. Springer-Verlag, Berlin 1977.

many participants who suffer from familial hypercholesterolemia, the inborn disease of very high cholesterol levels (above 350 dl/mg) that afflicts less than 1 percent of the population. Such people always have very high cholesterol values and often have severe vascular changes early in life. All of them will therefore be represented by symbols in the upper righthand corner of the diagram. If a study includes many of these people, along with people not afflicted with the disease, the statistics will be skewed and will automatically produce a correlation between high cholesterol levels and atherosclerosis. And if the written results of the study present only the mean statistical values and correlation coefficients, or if the symbols do not specify the participants with familial hypercholesterolemia, readers will not be able to discern this bias or skewing effect.

I shall not discuss here whether or not it is the high cholesterol that causes atherosclerosis in patients with familial hypercholesterolemia, or whether it is atherosclerosis that causes high cholesterol, or something else. What is certain, however, is that these people have a rare, genetic defect in their ability to metabolize cholesterol. For this reason, they cannot be used as proof that high cholesterol causes atherosclerosis in the remaining 99 percent of the population that is free of their disease. Individuals with familial hypercholesterolemia should be studied separately, as people with a biochemical problem of their own, not mixed in with people unaffected with the problem; that is elementary. Nevertheless, almost all studies include both groups. You may say that one percent of the population cannot have much influence on the result but in many studies, patients with familial hypercholesterolemia were heavily overrepresented. (See page 51.)

Thus, many factors can prevent a scientist from arriving at valid statistical calculations. Let's keep that fact in mind as we look at some of the studies that have convinced the scientific community that high cholesterol causes atherosclerosis.

Landé and Sperry

The first study designed to demonstrate a possible correlation between blood cholesterol and degree of atherosclerosis was published by the pathologist Kurt Landé and the biochemist Warren Sperry of the Department of Forensic Medicine at New York University.[2] The year was 1936. They studied large groups of individuals who had died violent deaths. To their surprise, they found absolutely no correlation between the amount of cholesterol in the blood and the degree of atherosclerosis. In age group after age group, their diagrams looked like the starry sky (Figure 4B).

Because Landé and Sperry were cautious and methodical, their study should have nipped the diet-heart idea in the bud. Or, more accurately, if those who promoted the diet-heart idea later on had read Landé and Sperry's paper before beginning their research, they would probably have dropped the idea at once.

But the few who remember Landé and Sperry misquote them and claim that they found a connection,[3] or they ignore their results by arguing that cholesterol values in the dead are not identical with those in the living.

Veterans explained away

That problem was solved by Dr. J. C. Paterson from London, Canada, and his team.[4] For many years they followed about 800 war veterans. These men were confined to a hospital because they were mentally ill or needed residential care. Over the years, Dr. Paterson and his co-workers regularly analyzed blood samples from the veterans. Because the veterans were all between the ages of 60 and 70 when they died, the scientists had good information about their cholesterol levels during the period of time when atherosclerosis normally develops.

Cholesterol levels varied considerably from one veteran to another, but for each individual it was fairly constant, so that, for example, those who had low cholesterol at the beginning of the study usually had low cholesterol just before they died. A post-mortem was performed on all the veterans who died and an atherogenic index was assigned to each individual, based on a visual, microscopic and chemical analysis of the coronary and central arteries. Like Drs. Landé and Sperry, Dr. Paterson and his colleagues did not find any connection between the athero-genic index and blood cholesterol levels; patients with low cho-lesterol were just as sclerotic as those with high cholesterol.

But the veteran studies were also explained away. Support-ers of the diet-heart idea declared that the veterans had eaten the same food, and that there are much greater variations in the amount of dietary fat consumed by people who do not live in an institution.

Although we don't know what each individual veteran ate, it is probably safe to assume that many supplemented the hos-pital diet with candy bars and potato chips and other suppos-edly unhealthy foods. And it is also probably a safe assumption that some of the veterans left the fattier foods untouched on their plates in the dining hall, whereas others did not. But let us as-sume that all these men ate approximately the same amount of fat, confined as they were to an institution. In that case, the diet-heart idea that blood cholesterol depends on the amount and type of fat we eat must be wrong, because the blood cholesterol levels of these veterans varied considerably, just as much as in the study by Landé and Sperry. (See Figure 4B.)

High cholesterol and smooth arteries

In the city of Agra in India, Dr. K. S. Mathur and his co-workers performed a similar study.[5] Their first step was to mea-sure blood cholesterol in 20 patients shortly before death and then a varying number of hours afterwards. They found that the cholesterol values were nearly the same if sampled before death and within 16 hours afterwards. Thus, blood samples taken very shortly after death are reliable—an important confirmation of the study done by Drs. Landé and Sperry. Dr. Paterson's group in

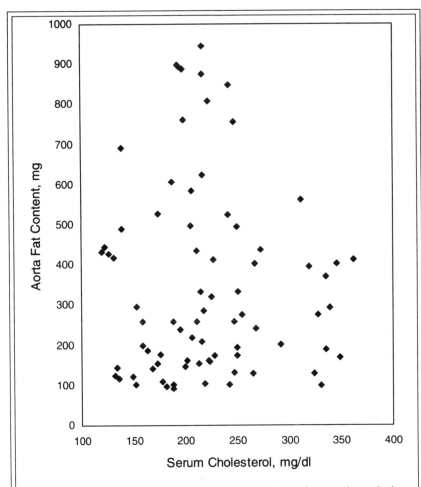

Figure 4B. Correlation between blood cholesterol and the lipid content of the aorta (a measure of atherosclerosis) in individuals between the ages of 30 and 59 who died suddenly. Data from Landé and Sperry.[2]

Canada did a similar test and obtained the same result.

Next, Dr. Mathur and his colleagues studied 200 people who had died in accidents, without any preceding disease. Like Drs. Landé and Sperry, and like Dr. Paterson, the Indian researchers could find no connection between cholesterol values and the degree of atherosclerosis. Those with low cholesterol had just as much atherosclerosis as those whose cholesterol was high.

Similar studies have also been performed in Poland,[6] in Guatemala[7] and in the US,[8] all with the same result: no correlation between the level of cholesterol in the blood stream and the amount of atherosclerosis in the vessels.

We are the only good ones

But some studies did find a correlation. One of these was the famous study from Framingham, Massachusetts, described in Chapter 2.

The correlation in Framingham was minimal, however. In statistical terms, the correlation coefficient was only 0.36. Such a low coefficient indicates a desperately weak relationship between variables, in this case, of course, between cholesterol and atherosclerosis. Usually, scientists demand a much higher correlation coefficient before they conclude that there is a biologically important relationship between two variables. Usually. . . but Framingham was not quite the usual case. It involved huge amounts of government funding.

Researchers arrived at the very low correlation coefficient only after much study. First, many of the townspeople of Framingham had their cholesterol tested several times over a period of several years. Then, Dr. Manning Feinleib of the National Heart, Lung, and Blood Institute led a team of co-workers in studying the coronary vessels of those who had died. The researchers were eager to learn which of the many factors they had studied was most important in the development of atherosclerosis in these dead people from Framingham. Was it blood cholesterol or the number of cigarettes smoked or something else?[9]

After carefully describing the atherosclerosis in the coronary arteries of the dead people, Dr. Feinleib and his associates concluded that it was blood cholesterol levels that best predicted the degree of atherosclerosis. Neither age nor weight nor blood pressure nor any other factor was as good as blood cholesterol, they said. But the correlation coefficient between cholesterol and atherosclerosis was a mere 0.36.

The study's written report offered no diagrams and no raw data about the cholesterol levels and degree of atherosclerosis of each of the individuals whose bodies had been examined. And the report did not discuss the low correlation coefficient; it didn't even comment upon the matter.

When scientists reach a result contrary to all others, it is routine—not merely usual but routine—to provide a detailed report about the result and also to discuss any possible ways in which the study may have been biased. In the Framingham study, there was an especially great need to follow this routine scientific procedure. Not only was the correlation coefficient trivial, but this study, funded with millions of taxpayer dollars by the National Institutes of Health, could have a major impact on national health care and the American economy. If there was no connection between cholesterol and atherosclerosis—as all the previous studies had shown—then there was no reason to bother about lowering cholesterol or changing the diet. Billions of taxpayer dollars could have been spent more wisely than in cholesterol-lowering measures for healthy people.

But the scientists conducting the Framingham study had no reservations. They were eager to stress their own excellence and to highlight the weaknesses of Dr. Paterson's Canadian war veterans study. In their report, they did not mention the studies of Drs. Landé and Sperry at all, nor the study of Dr. Mathur in India, nor the studies in Poland or Guatemala, nor the other US study. And when the Framingham study authors mentioned Dr. Paterson's study, it was only to criticize without putting their own cards on the table. Some of those hidden cards make for fascinating speculation.

For example, how were the dead of Framingham chosen for postmortem examination? From 914 deceased individuals, the researchers examined only 281. And from the 281, they selected 127 (14 percent of all who died) as subjects of the autopsy program for investigating the heart and its vessels.

Thus, those chosen for autopsy in the Framingham study were not a random sampling of the population, as they had been in the previous studies. The report from Framingham said nothing about the selection criteria, although scientific studies routinely do. Usually, the determining factor is age. A postmortem is seldom performed on people who have died peacefully in old age, as most of us will. Primarily, a postmortem is restricted to young and middle-aged people who have died before their time, and so it was in the Framingham study. Almost half of those autopsied were younger than 65 years. For this reason, the autopsied subjects must have included a relatively large number with familial hypercholesterolemia, the unusual genetic disease of cholesterol metabolism that prevents many of its victims from living to be 65. Furthermore, people with this disease are of special interest to scientists studying the cholesterol problem and were, therefore, with all certainty chosen for autopsy in a program tailored to investigate coronary disease. With only 14 percent of the Framingham dead chosen for autopsy, the risk of preferentially selecting those with this metabolic defect must have been great.

The ungrateful dead

Two studies with a design similar to that of the Framingham study were conducted in Japan. One, led by Dr. Noriya Okumiya, took place at Kyushu University;[10] the other, directed by Drs. Shuichi Hatano and Toshihisa Matsuzaki, took place at the Geriatric Hospital in Tokyo.[11] In both studies the researchers said that the level of blood cholesterol correlated with the degree of atherosclerosis.

But in the first of these autopsy studies, the correlation appeared only in people with a low or normal cholesterol level; in the second, it appeared only in elderly people. The reports of the studies presented no individual figures, merely correlation coefficients, and these were as small as those in the Framingham study. Moreover, the researchers did not explain the fact that the

small correlation coefficient between cholesterol and atherosclerosis was present only in some groups but not in others.

Even more remarkable, among the dead people with high
cholesterol, the degree of atherosclerosis was the same, whether
these people were young or old. Logically, since atherosclerosis
develops over time as people grow older, it should develop faster
in people whose cholesterol is high, at least it should if the diet-
heart idea were true.

Perhaps you're thinking that the degree of atherosclerosis
was the same in all age groups because death had consistently
weeded out only the most atherosclerotic. But all degrees of atherosclerosis were present among those who had died.

The fact that atherosclerosis was just as severe in people of
all ages with high cholesterol must mean that the cholesterol
level was unimportant. After all, if the cholesterol level had been
of any importance, the old people would have been much more
sclerotic than the younger ones, after living far longer with high
cholesterol.

Similar peculiar results turned up in a study done in Oslo,
Norway, where scientists have investigated atherosclerotic diseases for many years in studies involving a great number of the
city's inhabitants. The project included a study of coronary atherosclerosis, led by Dr. Lars Solberg and his co-workers, in cooperation with researchers at Louisiana State University in New
Orleans. In their final report, these authors claimed that in Oslo,
too, the degree of atherosclerosis correlated with the level of blood
cholesterol. But, as in the previous studies, the correlation was
weak. And the correlation may have stemmed from the fact that
the researchers did not consider the 20-year age difference between the youngest and the oldest of the people they studied.[12]

In the Oslo investigation, the weakness of the correlation
between atherosclerosis and cholesterol appeared in many ways.
For instance, many of the people with normal coronary vessels
had cholesterol levels as high as people for whom all three coronary vessels were constricted. Furthermore, people with two nar-

rowed coronary vessels had, on average, lower cholesterol levels than those with just one narrowed vessel. The scientific word for such results is "unsystematic," which means that Mr. Chance or Mrs. Bias have determined their outcome.

Coronary angiography

If we take a solution of iodine atoms and inject them into a blood vessel of a living person, we can see the inside of the vessel with x-rays. This is the principle behind the medical technique called angiography. A narrow and flexible plastic tube is inserted into the femoral artery in the groin and pushed gently upwards through the aorta, the chief artery of the human body, until it reaches the vessel to be investigated, such as the coronary vessels, those that provide the heart muscle with blood. When the tip of the catheter reaches the entrance of one of the coronary

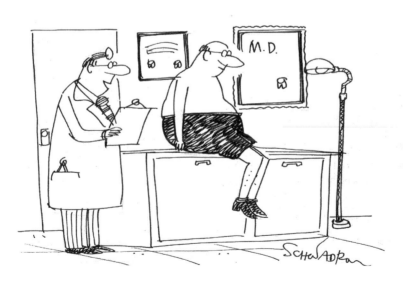

"Good news, Mr. Dewlap. While your cholesterol
has remained the same, the research findings have changed."

vessels, the iodine solution is slowly injected.

With the advent of bypass surgery, which allows us to re-place old and roughened coronary vessels with new and smooth ones, coronary angiography has gained great importance. On the x-ray pictures, shadows show how much the coronary vessels have been narrowed.

If we know the cholesterol values of patients with coronary angiography, and compare these values with their angiographic pictures, we can test the cholesterol hypothesis. If blood chole-sterol is the most important factor in the production of athero-sclerosis, as we have been told for decades, then people with rough and irregular vessel shadows should have higher choles-terol levels than people with smooth artery shadows.

It seems as though every specialist in coronary angiography in America has performed his own study, funded with federal tax monies awarded by the National Heart, Lung and Blood Insti-tute. In paper after paper published in various medical journals, using almost identical words, these medical specialists empha-size the importance of the blood cholesterol level for the develop-ment of atherosclerosis.[13]

But the reports offer no individual figures, only correlation coefficients, and these are never above a minimal 0.36, usually even smaller. And they never mention any of the previous studies that found no association between degree of atherosclerosis and level of blood cholesterol.

Studies based on coronary angiography are fundamentally flawed, at least they are if their findings are meant to be applied to the general population. Coronary angiographies are mainly performed on young and middle-aged patients with symptoms of heart disease, which means that a great number of patients with familial hypercholesterolemia are included in all angiographic studies so there is an obvious risk for the kind of bias that I have described earlier.

The fact that this objection is justified was demonstrated in a Swedish study performed by Dr. Kim Cramér and his co-workers in Gothenburg, Sweden. As in most other angiographic studies, the patients with the highest cholesterol values had, on average, the most sclerotic coronary vessels.

But if those who were treated with cholesterol-lowering drugs were excluded, and almost certainly this group must have included all patients with familial hypercholesterolemia, the correlation between blood cholesterol and degree of atherosclerosis disappeared.[14]

Risk factors and coronary vessels

The theory that the level of cholesterol determines whether atherosclerosis will appear or not also conflicts with results from a number of long-term angiographic studies of the coronary arteries. The aim of the studies was to explore which factors dictated the development of atherosclerosis. Were the risk factors primary or secondary? Should they be sought among the mercenary troops or were they something that followed the vestige of war, like hunger and cholera? Was smoking of any importance? Did blood pressure influence the development of atherosclerosis? Or was it high blood cholesterol?

According to conventional wisdom, atherosclerosis increases if the cholesterol is high over a long period of time or if it merely goes up, no matter why. Likewise, atherosclerosis decreases, or at least it should not increase, if cholesterol is low or if it goes down. An association between an increase in the suspected causal factor, in this case cholesterol, and a worsening of the disease, in this case atherosclerosis, is called dose-response or exposure-response. The presence of exposure-response—in which the change in the suspected causal factor and the change in the incidence of the disease both go in the same direction, and only in that direction—strongly supports the idea that the factor in question is causal. However, the presence of exposure-response is not sufficient to prove causality because an innocent risk marker may go in the same direction as the real cause and thus introduce a false impression of exposure-response. But absence of exposure-response definitely disproves causality. Studies of ex-posure-response are therefore of great importance.

One of the first who studied the inside of the coronary ves-sels with such questions in mind was Dr. Charles Bemis. The year was 1973. Together with his team at the Peter Bent Brigham Hospital in Boston,[15] he studied about 70 patients and found that the only factor that could be connected with the degree of atherosclerosis was the cholesterol level at the start of the inves-tigation. In patients with high blood cholesterol at the start, coro-nary atherosclerosis had increased at the following angiographic examination a couple of years later.

So far, the results were as anticipated. Once again, it was demonstrated that high blood cholesterol is a risk factor for coro-nary heart disease. Now to the interesting finding.

In 24 patients, cholesterol had decreased by more than 25 percent between the two angiographies, a lowering that was con-siderably greater than in most cholesterol-lowering trials. Among these 24 patients atherosclerosis had increased in 16, while it was unchanged in just eight. In 12 patients cholesterol had in-creased, but only four of them had increased atherosclerosis.

Put another way, two out of three whose cholesterol went down had become more sclerotic, while this was the case in only one out of three whose cholesterol went up. It should, of course, have been the other way around.[15]

Dr. Bemis' result was confirmed the following year by Dr. Demetrios Kimbiris and his group in Philadelphia.[16] These in-vestigators also found that cholesterol was unimportant. The coronary arteries of 17 out of 25 patients with high cholesterol had worsened, but they had also worsened in seven out of ten patients with low cholesterol.

Similar results were observed at the famous Mayo Clinic by Dr. Clarence Shub and his colleagues.[17] They found that coro-nary atherosclerosis had increased in all patients whose chole-sterol had decreased by more than 60 mg/dl, a reduction that should have been considered more than acceptable in any cholesterol-lowering trial.

Study after study has confirmed the startling finding of Bemis and his colleagues.[18] In their paper, Dr. John Kramer and his colleagues at the Departments of Cardiology and Biostatistics, the Cleveland Clinic Foundation, concluded: ". . . medical treatment directed toward 'secondary prevention' may be unsuccessful in retarding or reversing the development of progressive arterial lesions and their clinical consequences."[18c]

The fact that coronary atherosclerosis gets worse just as fast or faster when cholesterol goes down as when it goes up, the opposite of exposure-response, should have led scientists to question the whole diet-heart idea. But nobody did.

In 1993, a team led by Canadian researcher Dr. David Waters published yet another study. This one included 335 patients.[19] They found that when, after a two-year interval, the coronary vessels had narrowed by more than 15 percent, the risk for cardiac death or a nonfatal heart attack increased considerably. They concluded that the changes seen in coronary angiography were a good substitute for cardiac events in clinical trials.

What they neglected to note was that on average the cholesterol level of those whose atherosclerosis had progressed did not differ significantly from the cholesterol level of those whose atherosclerosis had not progressed. Here it should be mentioned that in the angiographic trials (see Chapter 6), the cholesterol level usually fell by 30-50 percent, whereas the change in vascular diameter was very small, less than one percent. In Waters' study the change in diameter was more than 15 percent, but the decrease in cholesterol was an insignificant 2 percent. Such results do not suggest that blood vessel diameter changes have anything to do with cholesterol changes.

You may think that I have selected only studies that did not demonstrate exposure-response. Perhaps the studies cited above are examples of bad science because bad science is so common. Perhaps I have overlooked studies of better quality that did demonstrate exposure-response. I have put that question to myself and, eager not to overlook any such studies, I made a systematic search for all studies that have recorded changes of the coronary artery system and at the same time recorded changes in total or LDL-cholesterol. After having examined several hundred studies, I found a total of 22 studies that satisfied my criteria—seventeen angiographic trials and five observational studies—some of which were mentioned above.[20] Except for one study, none of them found evidence for exposure-response. Interestingly, with one exception, no other risk factor was associated with the progression of atherosclerosis either, not body weight nor smoking nor good cholesterol nor any other blood lipid. The exception was two trials that found a significant inverse relationship between the amount of physical exercise and the degree of atherosclerosis growth.[20g,20m]

To illustrate the lack of exposure-response, let me comment briefly on the study that achieved the largest cholesterol lowering of them all.

LAARS,
the LDL-Apheresis Atherosclerosis Regression Study

This study from the Netherlands was conducted by Dr. Abraham A. Kroop and his co-workers from various institutions at the university hospitals in Nijmegen and Leiden.[20n] They studied 42 men, 32 of whom had familial hypercholesteremia. All had extensive coronary atherosclerosis and cholesterol levels of at least 312 mg/dl. All patients were treated with simvastatin (Zocord®), one of the new cholesterol-lowering drugs called statins. (For more on the statins, see page 200.)

Half the patients were also treated with LDL-apheresis, in which a patient's blood plasma circulates through a system that chemically takes away most LDL, and thus also LDL-cholesterol, but has no effect on HDL-cholesterol. By combining simvastatin with LDL-apheresis, a further lowering of cholesterol takes place. Thus, whereas LDL-cholesterol in patients treated with simvastatin alone was lowered by an average of 47 percent, it was lowered by 63 percent in the patients who had both treatments—from 303 to 115 mg/dl. With such large changes in blood cholesterol levels, the researchers were confident that they could not only retard the progression of atherosclerosis, but even reverse it.

But there was no measurable difference between the two groups! Nine patients in the apheresis-medication group and 11 patients in the medication-only group showed worsening of atherosclerosis while two and five respectively showed improvement. Even more disturbing, there was no correlation between the degree of cholesterol lowering and the angiographic changes in individual patients. Worsening or improvement was seen whether LDL-cholesterol and total cholesterol were lowered by large amounts or whether they were lowered by moderate amounts.

The lack of exposure-response, found again and again in the cholesterol-lowering trials—both with the old cholesterol-lowering drugs and the newer, more effective statin drugs—should stimulate researchers to ask the fundamental question: Is the cholesterol concentration important at all? Instead, the authors of the reports merely state that the initial or the on-trial cholesterol concentrations predict the outcome. Often they predict correctly, but this finding adds nothing to what we knew before the trial, namely that high cholesterol is a risk factor for CHD. To prove that high cholesterol is the villain—and not just an innocent bystander—demands that a *change* in the cholesterol concentration in each individual is followed by a *change* in degree of atherosclerosis in the same direction. But in all studies these changes occurred haphazardly.

Another Japanese paradox

You have already heard that the Japanese diet is Spartan compared to Western standards, their blood cholesterol is low and the risk of getting a heart attack in Japan is much smaller than in any other country. Given these facts you are justified in concluding that in Japan atherosclerosis is rare.

In the 1950s, Professors Ira Gore and A. E. Hirst at Harvard Medical School and Professor Yahei Koseki from Sapporo, Japan, studied the arteries of both American and Japanese individuals.[21] At that time the average blood cholesterol level for Americans was about 220 mg/dl whereas for the Japanese it was about 170 mg/dl.

Researchers looked at the aorta, the main artery of the body, in 659 Americans and 260 Japanese after death, meticulously recording and grading all signs of atherosclerosis. As expected, atherosclerosis increased from age 40 and upwards, both in Americans and in Japanese. Now to the shocking fact.

When the degree of atherosclerosis was compared in each age group, there was hardly any difference between Americans and Japanese. Between ages 40 and 60, Americans were a little more sclerotic than Japanese; between 60 and 80 there was practically no difference, and above 80, the Japanese were a little more sclerotic than Americans.

A similar study was conducted by Dr. J. A. Resch from Minneapolis and Drs. N. Okabe and K. Kimoto from Kyushu, Japan.[22] They studied the arteries of the brain in 1408 Japanese and in more than 5000 Americans and found that in all age groups Japanese people were *more* sclerotic than Americans.

Those who want us to lower our cholesterol say that heart attacks are caused by atherosclerosis in the coronary vessels, not in the aorta or the cerebral arteries, and they are right. Curiously, the coronary arteries of Japanese people are, in fact, less affected by atherosclerosis than the coronary arteries of Americans, and this may explain why the Japanese have heart attacks less often than Americans.

But why are the aorta and the arteries of the brain just as sclerotic in Japan where cholesterol is much lower than in the US? If high cholesterol causes atherosclerosis in the artery walls, it should, of course, do it in any artery because the cholesterol level is identical whether the blood comes from the heart or the brain or any other organ.

Isn't it much more likely that something else causes athero-sclerosis than cholesterol? Something that may vary between the arteries, such as blood pressure. Blood pressure may vary greatly in various arteries depending on their size and the tension of the smooth muscular cells in the vessel wall. For instance, the ten-sion of the coronary vessels, but not necessarily of other vessels, increases significantly when we are mentally stressed. Mental stress varies considerably between individuals and, as Dr. Marmot argued in his Japanese migrant study, probably also between populations.

Cholesterol is innocent

That people with low cholesterol become just as sclerotic as people with high cholesterol is, of course, a devastating blow to the diet-heart idea. But the names of Landé, Sperry, Paterson, and Mathur are absent in the hundreds of papers and books that the proponents publish every year.

"But what about the animal experiments?" they say. "You cannot explain away all the animal experiments!"

What animal experiments have taught us is the subject of the next chapter.

Myth 5

Animal Studies Prove the Diet-Heart Idea

Rabbit tricks are positive successes.
> Harry Houdini
> Hungarian-American magician (1874-1926)

Animals eat the wrong food

Perhaps you're finding that the cholesterol question in man is a little complicated—and it is. But it's nothing compared to the situation in the animal kingdom, although, if it will comfort you, I'll begin by saying that cholesterol studies in animals just don't apply to man.

When it comes to cholesterol, none of the other mammals is like us. They have other amounts of it in their blood, different dietary habits, and most of them do not become atherosclerotic.

Many mammals never eat food containing cholesterol. If they are force-fed a cholesterol-rich diet, the cholesterol level of their blood rises to values many times higher than ever seen in normal human beings. And since such animals cannot dispose of the cholesterol they have eaten, every organ soaks up the cholesterol like a sponge soaks up water.

If animals are so different from us, how can we use them to prove that high-fat food and cholesterol are dangerous to human beings? Using cholesterol-rich fodder, it is possible to induce arterial changes that vaguely resemble human atherosclerosis in rhesus monkeys, but it is not possible in baboons. How do we know whether man reacts like a rhesus monkey or like a baboon or in some other way?

These obvious weaknesses in the animal studies have not prevented thousands of scientists from thinking up numerous ways to test animals in their laboratories.

There are, however, many experiments and observations that may give us food for thought. Let's start by looking at atherosclerosis and coronary disease in wild animals. What does atherosclerosis look like in the arteries and hearts of animals living outside the laboratory?

Atherosclerosis similar to that in man has been found in many animals, but its appearance is less widespread, probably because many wild animals suffer violent deaths as youngsters and thus rarely reach the age of atherosclerosis. An animal with pronounced atheroscloersis may also be an easy prey.

Atherosclerosis is found most often in birds, possibly because their blood pressure is higher than that of land animals. But animal fat or cholesterol in the diet is not the cause. The seed- and grain-eating pigeons, for instance, and the fish-eating penguins become just as atherosclerotic as the birds of prey.

There is no support for the diet-heart idea from the four-legged creatures either. Atherosclerosis has not been observed in beasts of prey, but it is not unusual in the vegetarian mammals they devour. Sea lions and seals also become atherosclerotic; obviously it doesn't help them that their fish diet provides more polyunsaturated fat than most humans eat.[1]

Unfortunately, heart disease researchers have not shown much interest in the naturally occurring atherosclerosis in animals. For a scientist with an open mind, many relevant questions could serve as springboards for interesting research. For instance, if vascular changes similar to human atherosclerosis are found in some wild animals but not in others, why do these changes occur in the vegetarians and the sea animals and not in those feasting on animal fat? And is it possible to prevent or treat spontaneous atherosclerosis in animals?

Instead, most scientists have already decided that atherosclerosis is what appears when they force-feed laboratory rabbits with fat and cholesterol.

Let's have a look at some of their results.

Rabbits and cholesterol

The rabbit is a docile and placid animal. It doesn't bite, taking blood samples from its long ears is easy, and rabbits are
cheap. But the main reason that the rabbit has become the most
common animal in the cholesterol laboratories is because of the
way it reacts to cholesterol-rich fodder.

The rabbit, of course, is a vegetarian. If a rabbit is forced to
eat food that it would never eat voluntarily and that it cannot
digest or metabolize, its blood cholesterol rises to values ten to
20 times higher than the highest values ever noted in human
beings. Cholesterol percolates all through the rabbit; its liver and
kidneys become fatty, its fur falls out and its eyes become yellowish from a buildup of cholesterol that it can neither store nor
metabolize nor excrete. Finally, it dies, not from heart disease
but from loss of appetite and emaciation—it starves.

It is true that cholesterol is also deposited in the arteries of
the rabbit, but these deposits do not even remotely resemble those
found in human atherosclerosis. Cholesterol appears in different places in a rabbit's vessels than in man's, the microscopic
changes are different, no hemorrhages or clefts appear as they
do in man, and no thrombus or aneurysm formation in the artery wall is seen. The most striking fact is that it is impossible to
induce a heart attack in a rabbit by dietary means alone. The
only result of cholesterol-feeding that the rabbit shares with man
is increased cholesterol content of the arterial wall.

Overfeeding other beasts with cholesterol and animal fat
produces varying results. The characteristics of the pathologic
changes are similar to those in the rabbit, but the amount and
location of cholesterol in the arterial walls vary. As a rule, it is

extremely difficult to provoke a heart attack in animals by dietary manipulation. To be successful, the scientist needs to combine diet with something else, such as a hormone injection or mechanical damage to the animal's arteries.[2]

In rare experiments heart attacks have been seen in laboratory animals fed with cholesterol and animal fat. But this is no proof that the food is the cause, because both atherosclerosis and coronary heart disease occur in zoo animals fed their natural food. To prove that the unnatural food causes a heart attack, two groups of laboratory animals should be studied, with one group receiving the high-fat food and the other group receiving its natural food.

Hunger-striking hearts

Those who experiment with animals often forget that the animals don't like it. This fact is crucial in studies of coronary heart disease, since frustration and psychological stress are considered a possible cause of the disease. In this context it may be interesting to look at some experiments performed by the American physician and scientist Dr. Bruce Taylor and his co-workers. (This is the same Dr. Taylor we discussed in Chapter 1.) The diet-heart proponents often cite these experiments as proof that animal fat causes atherosclerosis and coronary heart disease in man.

Dr. Taylor and his colleagues studied wild rhesus monkeys captured from the jungle. To produce "atherosclerosis," they gave the monkeys fodder to which had been added huge amounts of cholesterol. Throughout the experiment, the monkeys were housed individually in small dog cages, an arrangement they obviously disliked. To prevent escape the cages were reinforced with solid metal sheets.

The monkeys liked their food even less than their housing. They ate little and threw the rest around their cages. For long periods they went on hunger-strikes.

Taking blood samples from these unhappy monkeys was

difficult for all involved. To get enough blood, the groin artery of the monkey was punctured, which the monkeys resisted violently—they screamed, urinated and defecated.[3]

Of 27 monkeys, one had a heart attack after being subjected to four years of experimentation in this basement laboratory in Chicago. Interestingly, the scientists reported that this animal was especially hyperactive and extremely nervous.[4]

They reported on this fact but didn't elaborate. Maybe factors other than high blood cholesterol could have caused the heart attack in this intelligent animal isolated for years in a small cage, fed a bad-tasting diet and regularly subjected to terrifying blood samplings. Could that be? We don't know. Taylor and his colleagues, and most others who have cited this study in later papers, consider the cause to be the food and the high cholesterol level, that and nothing else.

In these experiments, the cholesterol of the monkeys climbed to values as high as ever measured in human beings. But it was not the cholesterol level that determined the outcome. This fact was demonstrated in an interesting experiment by Dr. Dieter Kramsch and his co-workers at the Evans Department of Clinical Research and the Cardiovascular Institute in Boston.

Dr. Kramsch and his colleagues studied as many monkeys as Dr. Taylor did, but Dr. Kramsch's project separated them into three groups. One group received fodder natural to monkeys, and the two others received fodder with added butter and cholesterol. The group fed the normal fodder and one of the groups fed the enriched fodder sat in their cages, inactive, throughout the experiment. The third group was allowed to exercise.

Only the inactive monkeys fed the butter and cholesterol developed coronary atherosclerosis and coronary heart disease. But the monkeys that were allowed to exercise had wide, almost smooth coronary arteries, although their cholesterol was almost as high as that of the inactive monkeys![5]

Unfortunately, Dr. Kramsch and his team did not report what happened with the inactive monkeys fed their normal fodder.

This is most curious because had these monkeys *not* developed atherosclerosis, it would have meant that it is the combination of inactivity and high-fat food that produces atherosclerosis. And if these inactive monkeys on normal fodder *had* developed atherosclerosis just as did the inactive monkeys on high-fat fodder, it would have meant that inactivity, not high-fat food, is the culprit. Both alternatives would have added most interesting information. Could it be that the study results were so controversial that the researchers dared not report them? We don't know.

Honest proponents of the diet-heart idea admit that their hypothesis will be proven not by creating atherosclerosis and heart disease in animals, but by studying these problems in human beings. And they think they have successfully proven it. In the next chapter we shall see whether they are right.

Myth 6

Lowering Your Cholesterol
Will Lengthen Your Life

But besides real diseases we are subject to many that are only imaginary, for which the physicians have invented imaginary cures; these have then several names, and so have the drugs that are proper for them.

Jonathan Swift (1667-1745)

Time for truth

As one scientific study after another has shown, people can gorge on animal fat for many years and still keep their blood cholesterol low. What we have also learned is that atherosclerosis and heart attacks may occur whether one's food is rich or lean and, most surprisingly, whether one's blood cholesterol is high or low. Given these facts, is there any reason to think that heart attacks can be prevented by reducing blood cholesterol with diet or drugs?

Based on what I have presented so far, the answer is no. In fairness, however, it still may be possible that high-fat food contains something other than cholesterol and saturated fatty acids that might be dangerous to the heart; or that high blood cholesterol slows the coronary circulation in some way other than by stimulating atherosclerosis. It might just be possible to reach the correct conclusion from the wrong premises.

The diet-heart idea itself is invalid, as I have already demonstrated in several ways. But the best way to know for sure
whether high-fat food and high cholesterol levels are dangerous
is to use human beings as guinea pigs; to see whether coronary
heart disease can be induced by feeding these people animal fat
or by elevating their blood cholesterol; or to see whether heart
attacks can be prevented by feeding the experimental subjects a
low-fat diet or by lowering their blood cholesterol.

The idea of letting test subjects eat large amounts of animal
fat for several years must be rejected no matter how interesting it
seems because the ethical committees that approve all experiments on living creatures would certainly condemn the idea. For-
tunately, the Masai and other populations have already performed
the experiment for us with surprising results, as you know from
Chapter 1.

It is much easier to get permission for an experiment to lower
blood cholesterol. Many researchers have received permission
and have tried, although reducing blood cholesterol is possibly
more dangerous than increasing it, as I shall soon explain.

To evaluate the effect of lowering blood cholesterol, all other
risk factors must remain unchanged. If the test individuals also
stop smoking, reduce their body weight, start exercising, receive
treatment for their elevated blood pressure, change their jobs or
get fired, fall in love or get divorced, move to another place with a
different climate and culture or do something else that might
influence the condition of their heart or blood vessels, then we
will not know to which factor we should attribute the results. Is
it the cholesterol reduction or is it something else? And this is
not the only problem.

The diet-heart proponents say that the prevention of atherosclerosis cannot start too early in life. They add that the best
results may be seen if prevention starts before the rougher, more
rocky deposits develop in our arteries. Herein lies the problem,
however, because coronary heart disease is uncommon before
the age of 50. To prove that cholesterol reduction prevents heart

attacks in young and middle-aged people, it is therefore necessary to study many thousands of individuals, preferably those at
unusually high risk for heart attacks.

The question we ask is whether fewer heart attacks occur
among people whose cholesterol is lowered by treatment than
among untreated people. A cholesterol-lowering experiment must,
therefore, also include untreated control subjects. By control
subjects we mean people who have identical risk factors for coronary heart disease—people with, on average, the same blood
cholesterol, smoking habits, body weight and so forth as the individuals who will be manipulated with treatment.

In sufficiently large studies, risk factors usually become evenly
distributed by chance, provided that test subjects and control subjects are assigned to their two groups on the basis of a random
feature such as their day of birth, or by leaving their assignment to
a computer. Studies that include randomly selected control subjects are called controlled, randomized studies.

As you can see, it is extremely difficult to design even the
initial steps of a scientifically acceptable trial. The standards of
science are high, however. In fact, they are so high that, even if we
manage to select a test group and a control group with almost
identical risk factors for heart disease, we must remember that
almost identical and absolutely identical are not the same thing,
and that we will never know all the factors that may, or may not,
contribute to the development of the disease in these people.

To these inevitable problems the trial directors themselves
have added one more. In scientific experiments, it is crucial not
to vary more than one factor at a time. If the test individuals are
asked not only to lower their blood cholesterol but also to quit
smoking, to lose excess body weight, to exercise or to do something else that we think may be beneficial, then we will be unable
to determine whether a possible reduction in heart disease is
caused by cholesterol lowering or by something else. Unfortunately, this method, called "multiple risk factor intervention,"
has been used in many trials.

Sighted or blind?

Many researchers have tried to prevent coronary heart disease with diet or drugs. Some of the first trials had so many technical errors that even the diet-heart proponents ignore them when they argue for their idea in their reviews.

One of the more serious errors was that the trials were not blinded. For a trial to be blinded, the patients must not know whether they belong to the treatment group or to the control group. In the best experiments, called double-blind trials, not even the doctors know to which group any given patient belongs. Blindedness prevents the treated subjects from feeling better merely because they know they are being treated and the control subjects from feeling worse merely because they know they are receiving no treatment; double blindedness prevents the doctors who want the treated subjects to benefit from leaping to conclusions based more on their own hopes than on scientific facts.

Up to 1968, eleven dietary trials had been performed and reported to the research community. Professor Jerome Cornfield at the University of Pittsburgh and Dr. Sheila Mitchell at the National Heart, Lung and Blood Institute analyzed these trials. They found that the "best" results were obtained if the doctors knew to which group the participants belonged. In six trials, the doctors knew, and in four of these six the number of heart attacks was reduced. In five trials, the doctors did not know, and in three of these five there was no difference between the number of new heart attacks in the control and treatment groups; in one of these five trials, even more heart attacks and more deaths occurred in the treatment group than in the control group.[1]

Unfortunately, many of the trials that were conducted after 1968 were neither single nor double-blind, as we shall see.

Soybean oil against heart attacks

In the 1960s, Professor Jeremy Morris of London, England, led a team of physicians and scientists in an investigation to see whether the replacement of animal fat with soybean oil could have some preventive effect on coronary heart disease. This oil is rich in polyunsaturated fatty acids, those that are considered protective against atherosclerosis and coronary heart disease. Enrolled in the trial were about four hundred middle-aged men who had previously been admitted to four London hospitals because of a heart attack; half of these received a diet containing large amounts of soybean oil. (This is one of the few trials sponsored solely by a government, and not by a drug company or any other vested interest.)

When the researchers analyzed the results four years later, they could find no beneficial effects from using soybean oil. Although blood cholesterol had decreased considerably in the treatment group, 15 had died of a heart attack. In the control group, 14 had died; and the number of nonfatal heart attacks was identical for both groups.[2]

The authors of the report compared their result with a similar but unblinded experiment performed by Dr. Paul Leren, a Norwegian researcher from Oslo.[3] They concluded that, even if Dr. Leren had been more successful, the results of the two trials taken together showed that it was not possible to prevent heart attacks by consuming more polyunsaturated oils.

At about the same time, Dr. Seymor Dayton and his team from the University of California at Los Angeles conducted a similar trial, the Veterans Administration trial.[4] At a nursing home for war veterans, they gave a treatment group of four hundred men a diet rich in soybean oil; the four hundred control subjects ate the institution's usual diet. Great efforts were made to prevent both patients and doctors from knowing who was treated and who was not.

Seven years later, a slightly smaller number of those who had eaten the soybean-oil diet had died from a heart attack. But the lower number of heart attack deaths was balanced by a higher number of cancer deaths.

Moreover, when the researchers analyzed the degree of atherosclerosis and the amount of cholesterol and fat in the arteries of the dead subjects, they discovered something peculiar. Although blood cholesterol had been lowered in the treatment group, the investigators found no difference between the degree of atherosclerosis in either group. In fact, a postmortem showed that those who had eaten the diet high in soybean oil had even more cholesterol in the aorta, the chief artery of the arterial system, than those who had eaten the nursing home's standard fare.

The report from this well-designed trial did not explain why mortality from atherosclerotic vascular disease had decreased but atherosclerosis itself had not. The authors of the report concluded that the effect of the trial was impressive, but that the trial alone was not enough to prove the diet-heart idea; it could not be used as an argument for recommending dietary changes for the entire population, since only old men had been studied and total mortality had not been lowered. The authors could also have said that the number of heavy smokers was much higher, indeed significantly higher according to the statistical tests, in the control group. Because smoking is considered a cause of coronary heart disease, the greater number of heart attacks in the control group could, logically, have resulted from smoking and not from the diet.

The reports from this trial are unusually sensible. It is difficult to find such balanced views from the directors of the trials that were to come.

The Coronary Drug Project

Blood cholesterol can be lowered in many ways. But which way is the most effective, and does it really help? These were the main questions needing answers when the American government's National Heart, Lung and Blood Institute started the first mammoth trial to lower blood cholesterol. The year was 1967.

The trial, headed by professor Jeremiah Stamler from Chicago, was called the Coronary Drug Project. It was designed to test four drugs—nicotinic acid, clofibrate (Atromidin®), thyroid hormone and estrogen (the female sex hormone), the latter given in two different dosages. Because these drugs and hormones lower blood cholesterol, researchers considered them appropriate for efforts to prevent coronary heart disease.

The Coronary Drug Project included more than 8000 middle-aged men who had already had at least one heart attack. About 5500 of these men were randomly assigned to five treatment groups, with the rest assigned to a control group of roughly 2800. Altogether 53 hospitals, from regions covering the whole United States, contributed patients to this massive study.

The trial was well prepared and well funded. In the paper describing the project, six pages were devoted to the names of the researchers who were to study anything of interest to the subject of coronary heart disease.[5]

Within 18 months after the start of the trial, treatment for those who had received the high dosage of estrogen was discontinued because the hormone was causing heart attacks instead of preventing them. Furthermore, the patients were reluctant to continue taking the estrogen because they became impotent and developed feminine-looking breasts. The investigators concluded that "the potential value of this level of estrogen medication is probably limited."

Those who were treated with half the dose of estrogen continued the treatment,[6] but a few months later even the smaller dosage was found to be unfavorable. In addition to the side effects cited above, there were also more new cases of cancer.[7]

Treatment with thyroid hormone was discontinued as well. Although thyroid hormone lowered blood cholesterol, the treatment seemed to induce heart attacks instead of decreasing them, just as was the case with estrogen.[8] The remaining groups continued to the end of the trial.

The results after seven years were disappointing. Those who were treated with clofibrate had just as many deaths as those in the control group, and many of them suffered serious side effects from the treatment.[9]

Those receiving nicotinic acid suffered from even more side

effects. Almost all complained of flushing or skin rashes, half complained of itching, and one in five had stomach pains, nausea or other symptoms pertaining to the stomach and bowels. Other common side effects included gout (a painful inflammatory disease of the joints), burning pains while urinating, excessive sweating, serious disturbances of the heart rhythm and various skin diseases.[10] As the directors of the experiment wrote in their report: "Great care and caution must be exercised if this drug (nicotinic acid) is to be used for treatment of persons with coronary heart disease."

What they left unsaid, though, was how to exercise "care and caution." And how can we? How are we doctors to know, before treatment begins, who will experience side effects? The drug was ineffective, anyway, in preventing fatal heart attacks. And why should we use an ineffective drug?

Doctors still use nicotinic acid for prevention of coronary heart disease because of a peculiarity that appeared in a study years after the Coronary Drug Project ended.[11] Eight to nine years after all the treatment subjects stopped taking nicotinic acid, a follow-up study showed that fewer of them had died from a heart attack and fewer of them had died of any cause.

This result—no benefits from the drug during the trial, but fewer deaths years later—stimulated much speculation. Perhaps the nasty side effects of nicotinic acid had concealed its positive effects during the trial. Researchers wondered whether it took many years before measures to lower blood cholesterol showed positive results. If so, the disappointing results of other trials should also be revisited.

Clofibrate had lowered blood cholesterol just as much as nicotinic acid had during the trial yet the drug prevented no deaths after the passage of many years. In fact, as the years passed, the number of fatal heart attacks in the group that had once received this drug was a little greater than in the control group. And nobody mentioned the follow-up findings of another large experiment, the WHO trial (described later), in which more people died from heart attacks four to five years after their treatment with clofibrate ended than those in the control group.

It seems strange that a drug could help years after being discontinued, as strange as if aspirin taken unsuccessfully to relieve a headache on Monday could prevent a headache the following Friday.

It is difficult to draw any conclusions from the cholesterol-lowering trials. Sometimes cholesterol lowering results in fewer deaths from heart attacks; sometimes the same degree of lowering results in more deaths. Sometimes the benefit is seen after a short time, sometimes not until years after trial's end. Or, if there is no benefit—the most common result—the trial directors declare that if the trial had continued longer, there might have been some benefit. However, when trials are sometimes beneficial and sometimes not, the most likely conclusion is that they aren't effective at all, and that their outcome depended on chance.

Primary versus secondary

The trials we have discussed so far are examples of secondary prevention. "Secondary" means that a disease—coronary heart disease, in this instance—has already occurred, and that treatment is aimed at halting further occurrence of the disease. In contrast, a treatment aimed at preventing the disease in apparently healthy people is called a "primary" prevention trial.

There is a fundamental difference between primary and secondary prevention. Very often, people who have already had a heart attack are badly frightened and ask themselves, "Will I survive another one?" To prevent another heart attack, many are willing to submit to rather unpleasant kinds of treatment. Healthy people whose only "defect" is high cholesterol are less inclined to exercise, to renounce cigarettes and good food and, above all, to take expensive drugs with unpleasant side effects. Healthy people thus make less compliant treatment subjects in a trial.

In addition, to achieve significant results, a primary prevention trial requires many more subjects, because the risk of a heart attack is considerably smaller for people who have never had one than for those who have. While the subjects needed for a secondary prevention trial number in the hundreds, those needed for a primary prevention trial number many thousand. And if it is not possible to prevent a heart attack in those who have already had one, it is obviously more difficult to do so in healthy individuals. But, of course, the number of potential customers and the economic prospects for drug companies are much, much larger if primary prevention were proven to be possible.

However, the results of the primary prevention trials have not been any more successful than those of the secondary preventive trials, even if the diet-heart proponents say otherwise. But now it is up to you, the reader, to judge for yourself.

The Upjohn trial

In the early 1970s, Dr. Albert Dorr and his co-workers at the Upjohn Company, a large pharmaceutical manufacturer in Kalamazoo, Michigan, started a trial to test Upjohn's new cholesterol-lowering drug colestipol (Lestid®).

At a large number of hospitals in the US, doctors selected more than 2000 men and women with high cholesterol. In defiance of proper trial protocol, the patients were not randomly assigned to treatment and control groups. Instead, the local doctors consulted the directors of the Upjohn trial. With the results of the participants' blood analyses in hand, Upjohn's scientists decided which patients would receive the drug and which would receive an ineffective sugar pill, the placebo.

To assign participants of a trial in this way obviously introduces bias, especially when those who assign them have a vested interest in the results. As you will see, the distribution of risk factors in the treatment and control groups was far from even.

Two years later the results were analyzed. No effect was seen for the women in the trial. But the effect for the men was amazing. After only two years, the number of heart attacks for the men in the treatment group had been cut in half. Such remarkable results have never been achieved in any trial before or since.[12]

There was a snag, however. The blood analyses performed at Upjohn's laboratories showed that in the control group, the number of individuals with familial hypercholesterolemia, the inborn error of cholesterol metabolism, was greater than in the treatment group; the exact number was not given, however.[13] As you now know, the prognosis for these people is much worse than for others; many of them die young from a heart attack. It is not unreasonable, therefore, to suspect that large numbers of at-risk individuals in the control group may well have been the reason Upjohn derived such favorable results for its drug.

The WHO trial

At the same time a similar trial was under way, conducted under the auspices of the World Health Organization. This trial, led by Professor Michael Oliver at the University of Edinburgh, Scotland, also tested clofibrate.

For the WHO trial, researchers analyzed blood cholesterol in 30,000 healthy, middle-aged men in Edinburgh, Prague and Budapest. The men with the highest blood cholesterol levels were selected for the treatment, a total of 10,000 individuals. Half of them were treated with clofibrate, the other half with an ineffective placebo.

After about five years of treatment, 174 of those who had been taking the placebo had suffered a nonfatal heart attack, but only 131 of those treated with clofibrate. Apparently the drug was a success.

But the number who had *died* from heart attacks was equal. Worse yet, considerably more of those who had been treated with the drug had died from other diseases. In all three cities, more men in the treatment group had died. Taken together, 128 died in the clofibrate group and 87 in the placebo group. And four to five years after the trial, even the number of heart attack deaths was larger in the treatment group.[14] Yet clofibrate is still recommended in many countries as a useful drug.

Fat food and fit Finns

One of the nations with the highest mortality from coronary heart disease is Finland. The mortality is especially high in the province of North Karelia, for reasons unknown. The coronary mortality rate increased year by year up to the 1960s. Of course, the Finnish health authorities were concerned. To them, it was self-evident that the cause was high cholesterol, because in Finland cholesterol levels are higher than anywhere else, and some of the highest values are found in North Karelia.

A team of doctors and scientists headed by Professor Pekka Puska at the university in Kuopio decided to do something about the problem. They chose to start in North Karelia. To see whether their efforts were beneficial, they used the district of Kuopio as their control, because people in Kuopio died just as often from heart attacks as the people of North Karelia did and their cholesterol was equally high.

In 1972, a public health campaign began throughout North Karelia. Its aim was to prevent heart disease by focusing on smoking, high-fat food and high blood pressure. The message was proclaimed in the mass media, on posters, at public meetings and through campaigns in schools and work places. In Kuopio people were allowed to live as they had traditionally lived—with no advertising campaigns and no intervention.

Five years later the number of heart attacks among North Karelian men had decreased from 0.77 to 0.63 percent each year. The total mortality had also decreased. Leaders of the campaign were confident that the trend would show continued improvement in cardiovascular mortality.[15]

There was a problem, however. In Kuopio, where the inhabitants served as control subjects, the number of heart attacks had decreased even more, among women as well as men, although they ate and smoked as they had before. In fact, heart mortality had decreased in all the provinces of Finland (Figure 6A).

The disappointment of the campaign leaders is easy to imagine. All their enthusiasm and work were of no use. On the other hand, negative results can be and are most interesting for those whose curiosity is intact and who are more interested in knowledge than in the defense of old positions.

Two conclusions may be drawn from the results of the campaign. First, it could not have been high-fat food or smoking or high blood pressure that caused the many heart attacks in North Karelia. If it had been, the number of heart attacks should have

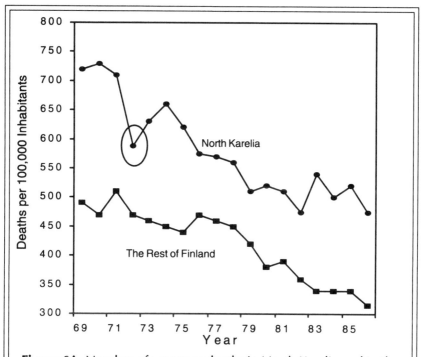

Figure 6A. Number of coronary deaths in North Karelia and in the rest of Finland. The circle indicates the starting point of the North Karelia project. Observe that more died from heart attacks during the first three years of the project than during the year before the start, most probably a result of chance. Seen over a longer period of time, heart mortality declined in North Karelia as well as in all of Finland and in many other countries. This decline had already started before the start of the North Karelia project. From Puska.[15]

decreased more in North Karelia than in untreated Kuopio. Second, something had happened in the whole country to cause coronary heart disease to decrease, and it was not an improved diet, it was not reduced smoking, and it was not a greater attention to blood pressure.

Unfortunately, the Finnish campaign team did not understand that they had found a track worth examining more closely. Instead, they published more papers with further analyses of their results. More had died in North Karelia during the campaign than in Kuopio, they agreed, but in North Karelia there had been a greater reduction in the number of heart attacks than in all other areas of Finland. They also thought that the small irregularities of the mortality curve for North Karelia proved that their campaign had been of benefit.[16]

But what they did not mention was that the decrease in heart mortality had started several years before the campaign had begun, and that an examination of the curve over a longer period of time clearly revealed that the campaign had made no impact. In fact, if the small irregularities in the curve had any significance at all, heart mortality in North Karelia had *increased* during the first three years of the campaign. (See Figure 6A.) But investigators were so convinced of their success that they started similar campaigns in other parts of Finland.

One of the campaign leaders, Dr. Jukka Salonen, had a differing opinion. In a letter to *The Lancet,* the famous medical journal, he explained that, although he was a co-author of the North Karelia report, he had not been able to read the paper with its optimistic conclusions before its publication! He did not think it possible to draw the conclusions presented in the paper and admitted that the steeper slope of the mortality curve for North Karelia could be explained in a variety of ways. For instance, he wrote, the increase in heart disease seen during the previous decades had come later to North Karelia; the decrease, therefore, had come later, too. The critical factor, however, was whether the campaign had changed the trend in North Karelia (which it had not). Dr. Salonen wrote that the North Karelia project could not be used as evidence to say that the risk factors either caused or did not cause heart disease; the project had merely shown that intervention is possible and can lead to a change in risk factors.[17]

But Professor Michael Oliver of Edinburgh (see Chapter 9) replied to Dr. Salonen's objections as follows: "What was the aim of trying to change risk factors unless they were thought to have some causative role and unless positive results were expected?"[18]

Valio

I am often asked why the producers of animal food have not reacted to the unscientific slander of their products. Let me describe what happened when some of the Finnish producers tried.

On June 23, 1988, a full-page advertisement appeared in a great many Finnish newspapers. The ad had been paid for by Valio, a large farm cooperative that markets about 90 percent of all milk products in Finland. The ads presented "five facts about dietary fat you have wished to hear about but nobody has told you." The five facts were as follows:

1. In Finland people eat less fat than in many Western European nations.
2. There is no direct connection between a nation's intake of animal fat and its mortality from coronary heart disease.
3. Fat intake and mortality from coronary heart disease have changed in opposite directions in many countries.
4. Mortality from coronary heart disease has decreased in Finland, despite the fact that the Finnish people have increased their consumption of animal fat.
5. Finally, the ad presented a short summary of the North Karelia campaign.

It would be an understatement to say that the director of Valio's research department, Kari Salminen, met stormy weather; it was more like a hurricane. He was attacked in all Finnish newspapers and journals; almost every day during that summer and autumn, critical editorials, articles and letters appeared in the Finnish press. No one could point to anything incorrect in the advertisement. Rather, journalists attacked the morality of the corporation. They condemned the advertisement as biased, misleading and unethical and charged that Valio had selected convenient statistics for a deliberate manipulation of scientific data.

As director of the North Karelia project, Professor Pekka Puska was particularly offended. He argued that the various efforts of the campaign had produced marked effects at the start. In this he was correct—except that the effects were in the wrong

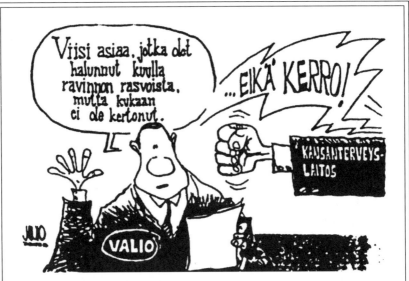

The Valio Man: Five facts about dietary fat you wanted to know but nobody told you. . .
The Fist (The Institute of Public Health): . . . and which you are not allowed to tell!

(Courtesy Jonko Innanen in the Finnish newspaper *Iltalehti*, July 1, 1988)

The public in Finland does not yet know that the North Karelia project was a failure. For many years its director, Pekka Puska, appeared in Finnish advertisements for margarine.

direction. The connection between dietary animal fat and heart disease has been better proved than most subjects in medicine, he wrote. The facts in the advertisement, he declared, did not tell the whole truth.

Kari Salminen, Valio's research director, answered that the advertisement had been designed as an invitation to debate and did not pretend to represent the whole truth.[19]

The invitation was ignored. Debate was replaced by execution.

The Oslo trial

In Oslo, Norway, Dr. Ingvar Hjermann and his team thought that smoking and high cholesterol levels were the two most important causes of coronary heart disease, and they wondered what would happen if smoking was stopped and blood cholesterol was lowered with an appropriate diet. To this end they studied about 1200 middle-aged men, mostly smokers, with high cholesterol. Half of these men received dietary advice and were encouraged to quit smoking. The rest received no treatment.

The Oslo trial results after five years appeared promising.[20] In the group given dietary and smoking advice, 19 died from a heart attack. In the control group, the number was 35; if, to the latter group was added a further control participant who had died suddenly of an unknown cause, the difference between the treatment and control groups became statistically significant.

It was a promising result for the diet-heart supporters. But did the experiment really prove that a faulty diet causes coronary heart disease?

In their paper, the Norwegian researchers pointed to two types of intervention, diet and cessation of smoking. They admitted that if dietary advice had been the only treatment, their result would not have been sufficient as evidence.

In fact, they had used three types of intervention, because subjects in the treatment group were also advised to lose weight. Evidently, this advice was followed because at the end of the trial, the mean weight difference between the two groups was almost seven kilograms (about 15 pounds).[21] Opinions vary as to the importance of a six-to-seven-kilogram weight difference. It is evident that the risk of diabetes and high blood pressure is greater for overweight people, and diabetes and high blood pressure predispose for coronary heart disease. Most proponents of the diet-heart idea also recognize overweight as a problem in heart disease. Wrote Dr. William Kannel, director of the Framingham project: "Avoidance and correction of obesity deserve a high priority among measures taken to avoid coronary heart disease, since the combined effect of the risk factors it promotes on coronary heart disease incidence is formidable."[22]

Now to the crucial question. Which of the measures had made the decisive effect in the Oslo trial? Was it lowering of cholesterol by diet, was it reduced smoking or was it weight loss? Nobody knows.

Possibly you're asking, "Why didn't the Oslo trial leaders concentrate on the diet alone?" The answer to that question can be found in a paper published earlier.

About ten years before the Oslo trial, the researcher who had performed the Norwegian soybean trial, Dr. Paul Leren, had published the latest results of that study. Although the number of heart attacks was reduced a little, Dr. Morris and his colleagues in England, using a similar treatment, had failed to reduce the number of heart attacks.[23] But Dr. Leren analyzed his own result and found that it might have been a good idea to change more than one risk factor, an approach called multiple risk factor intervention, because diet alone was unsuccessful.

Few of the diet-heart supporters rely on diet alone in their trials; instead they combine diet with other measures. When the massive Lipid Research Clinics trial was in the planning process (discussed on page 166), the scientists stated frankly that diet alone was not enough to lower cholesterol—cholesterol-lowering drugs were also necessary.[24]

It is laudable to try to prevent disease and premature death as effectively as possible. If all the measures are proven to be beneficial, the frontier should, of course, be broadened. But when various intervention measures are combined in one study, it is not possible to judge the influence of each measure individually. As no one has proved that diet alone is efficient, it would perhaps have been wiser to exclude dietary advice from the studies—or to study dietary changes alone.

MRFIT—Much ado about nothing

For many years scientists at the National Heart, Lung and Blood Institute had discussed how to prevent heart attacks. But before telling the American public what to do, they needed solid proof that their advice would work.

They had rejected the idea of using diet alone. To be successful, they said, it was necessary to attack at least three of the major risk factors: high cholesterol, smoking and elevated blood pressure. To this end the institute designed a gigantic trial called the Multiple Risk Factor Intervention Trial—MRFIT ("Mister Fit") for short.[25] At its head, once again, was Professor Stamler from Chicago.

The first step was to recruit more than 360,000 middle-aged men from eighteen American cities. After a routine investigation, the researchers selected about 12,000 men, namely those who were considered especially prone to heart attack.

The trial had every chance of success. The test subjects had entered the trial voluntarily, and they knew that their condition was considered dangerous. Although they felt hale and hearty (and, by normal standards, they were healthy), they were overweight, their blood pressure was too high and, according to the experimenters, their cholesterol scores hinted at premature death from heart disease. After the initial analyses, the men took part "with remarkably enthusiastic response."

However, one of those initial analyses should have stopped the whole MRFIT trial.

A decade before, a smaller test study had been conducted

with great care. A comparison of the food eaten by the men in this study with the food consumed by the men selected for MRFIT revealed that the MRFIT participants had eaten more "healthfully" in all respects, more in accord with the diet-heart idea.[26] Yet the blood cholesterol of the MRFIT participants was higher!

Furthermore, initial surveys indicated that those MRFIT participants who ate less saturated fat and cholesterol tended to have higher blood cholesterol! It was not exactly an encouraging finding for researchers who hoped to lower blood cholesterol by lowering dietary saturated fat and cholesterol. But the directors of the trial responded by declaring that cholesterol and saturated fat should be reduced more than originally planned for the MRFIT treatment group. Furthermore, they speculated that the fact that blood cholesterol was highest among the MRFIT subjects who ate the most "prudent" diet showed that these men must have changed their diet at the last minute, right before the trial began.

Perhaps the directors were correct. The participants could have made eleventh-hour dietary changes in the days just before they were questioned about what they ate. But when scientists are presented with experimental results contrary to what they have expected, they usually want to know "What's going on here? And why?" In accord with the long tradition of scientific inquiry, most scientists would have asked the MRFIT participants whether they really had shifted to a new diet right before the trial began. More than one hundred million dollars of taxpayers' money could have been saved if some scientists had asked that question. If MRFIT participants were eating as they had always eaten, even just before the trial, they would have demonstrated that diet is not an important factor in determining the cholesterol level, and this enormously costly trial could have been cancelled then and there.

But no one asked. Or did they? Perhaps it would have been too heroic for the directors to cancel a trial with all these doctors, nurses, dieticians and, most of all, the trial directors themselves lined up and assured that they would have lucrative and prestigious jobs for the next several years? If anyone asked, he didn't do it in public, and the trial continued.

The subjects were randomly assigned to two groups of equal size. Those placed in the treatment group and their families met in small groups to learn about the rationale behind the trial, and then, with the aid of dieticians, to learn how to read food labels, to choose low-fat foods in the grocery store, to cook with minimal fat and to change old recipes to meet new guidelines. The stated aim of the dietary advice was to reduce the men's intake of cholesterol and saturated fat and increase their intake of polyunsaturated fat.

The treatment subjects also met for an intensive antismoking campaign; in selected cases, even hypnosis was used to help participants quit smoking. When necessary, individual counseling was provided by doctors, nutritionists, psychologists, nurses and other health professionals. Every four months the treatment subjects were called in for blood sampling and for "counseling" sessions to determine whether they had fully understood all the new guidelines.

High blood pressure was treated energetically, and subjects with weight problems were taught how to reduce calories and get more exercise. Dieticians checked yearly to make sure that the men were really eating as prescribed.

The men in the control group received no advice, but they visited the center once a year for blood sampling and a questionnaire about their eating habits, and the results of these investigations were sent to their own doctors.

After seven years of treatment the results were analyzed. The trial directors were satisfied that there had been major risk-factor changes. Blood pressure had been lowered considerably, and many of the men had quit smoking. But blood cholesterol had decreased by only seven percent. It had decreased in the control group, too, although the control subjects had scarcely changed their diet at all, so the difference between the two groups was only two percent. Other risk factors had changed in the control group, as well. The one difference between the groups worth mentioning was that more of the control subjects continued to smoke.

The difference in number of deaths between the two groups was small. In the treatment group 115 had died of coronary heart disease, in the control group 124. According to statistical precepts, such a small difference could well have been due to chance. There was no statistical difference, either, in the number of deaths from all causes: 265 in the treatment group, 260 in the control group.[27]

Customarily, when a scientific experiment does not produce results supporting a hypothesis, the scientists admit it immediately. But this was not an ordinary experiment. More than a decade of hard work and several hundred millions of dollars had been invested in what was the most ambitious medical study ever conducted. Hundreds of doctors, professors, statisticians, dieticians, psychologists and others had participated. More than fifty scientific reports, most of them mammoth, had been published. And thousands of apparently healthy men and their families had been persuaded to take part in time-consuming investigations and to change their diet and way of life for many years.

This huge effort could not possibly have been in vain. And what had been preached for years to the American public about risk factors and heart attacks could not possibly have been wrong.

With a little statistical manipulation, the trial directors improved their results. Although not part of the original study design, the researchers decided to divide the participants into smaller groups. When the researchers excluded a subgroup that had particularly negative results, their overall result appeared better. Almost all the other subgroups had fewer fatal heart attacks by a slight margin—not all subgroups, but almost all.

This after-the-fact statistical manipulation permitted the trial directors to conclude that the MRFIT intervention program might have had a favorable effect for most of the participants. It was obvious, for example, that the outcome was favorable for those who had quit smoking. (In fact, subgroup analyses showed that cessation of smoking was the only intervention that had any effect on the outcome.[28])

It was less obvious that treatment of high blood pressure contributed to improved life span. In some of the subgroups, those taking drugs to lower blood pressure had more heart attacks, although in another subgroup treated with such drugs, the outcome was better.

Within four years after the end of MRFIT, a total of 202 men in the treatment group and 226 in the control group had died from heart disease; again a difference that could be explained by chance (or by changes in smoking habits). But the investigators claimed that the figures proved the benefit of lowering blood cholesterol.[29]

Diet-heart supporters who are more conservative admit that MRFIT was a failure, but they usually add that the failure occurred because blood cholesterol levels were lowered by a mere two percent, and that is too small to have any effect.

This is a reasonable objection. The change in blood cholesterol levels was trivial, even though the treatment group had embraced drastic dietary changes. They had cut their intake of cholesterol by almost half, they had lowered their intake of saturated fat by more than 25 percent and they had eaten 33 percent more polyunsaturated fat while the control group's diet was practically unchanged.[30] The inevitable conclusion is that diet is worthless as a preventive measure—a conclusion that could not be endorsed by MRFIT's directors.

If a scientific trial with almost unlimited funding and personnel cannot lower cholesterol more than two percent over seven years, how is the overworked general practitioner to succeed with a crammed waiting room and with no dieticians or experts in behavior modification to hold his hand? And how is the patient to be motivated if he can expect no rewards for all his trouble?

What MRFIT demonstrated is that it is a good idea to quit smoking. But we already knew that, and most people can manage to quit smoking without such costly help from officious health professionals. (Read more about MRFIT on page 50.)

The "final proof"—the Lipid Research Clinics Trial

Diet-heart proponents claim that if we had a drug that could lower blood cholesterol sufficiently without any serious side effects, we could prevent or at least delay all diseases caused by atherosclerosis.

This is a dream come true for doctors. All that's necessary to prevent heart disease is a prescription pad and a gadget for measuring cholesterol—and no time-consuming fuss with diet counseling.

And what a bonanza for the drug producers! A lifelong lowering of cholesterol with expensive drugs in a substantial portion of the population. The profits derived from brief penicillin treatments pale in comparison. Drug manufacturers calculated the profits in the billions of dollars.

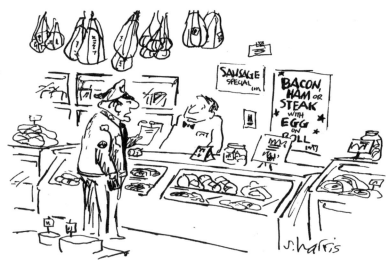

I'm from the cholesterol police
and I'd like a word with you.

Large trials using clofibrate had not been especially encouraging, to say the least. But other, newer drugs seemed more promising. One of them was cholestyramine (Questran®).

The National Heart, Lung and Blood Institute embarked on a new jumbo trial,[31] called The Lipid Research Clinics Coronary Primary Prevention Trial (LRC), to test the effectiveness of cholestyramine. The MRFIT trial had excluded men with extreme cholesterol values (above 350 mg/dl), as it was considered unethical to place such "patients" in a control group without treatment. In the LRC, all individuals with high cholesterol were included. The higher the cholesterol, the better.

To solve the "ethical dilemma" of lowering cholesterol in only half the patients, both the LRC's treatment group and the control group received dietary advice. Although this advice would lessen the difference in outcome between the two groups, the degree of cholesterol lowering from diet was expected to be insignificant! The great difference would be created by cholestyramine.

To find about 4000 test individuals, blood cholesterol was measured in almost one-third of a million middle-aged men. Never in history had so many people with such high blood cholesterol levels been involved in a medical experiment. In MRFIT the upper three percent of the cholesterol range was selected, but men with the highest values were excluded. In the LRC trial, only the upper 0.8 percent participated, without exception. Consequently, the mean blood cholesterol before the dietary treatment started was about 40 mg/dl higher than in MRFIT.

As in MRFIT, all LRC participants were thoroughly investigated. After a few weeks of dietary indoctrination, half of the men were started on cholestyramine medication while the other half received a supposedly inactive placebo powder.

Seven to eight years later, the results were analyzed. Although blood cholesterol in the treatment group had decreased by more than 8 percent, the differences in the numbers of heart attacks were so small that they could only be attributed to chance. Of those who had taken cholestyramine, 10 percent, or 190 men,

INSIDER INSIGHTS

"A final lesson worth noting is that the current cholesterol campaign represents a rare concordance of interests on the part of many constituencies. The health professions, the pharmaceutical industry, government, the public—all should benefit from efforts to promote and implement the recommendations and guidelines in the Adult Treatment Panel report. Physicians will benefit because they will be providing better medical care to their patients and incidentally will have available a new and expanded market of patients for preventive medical care. The pharmaceutical industry will benefit from the greatly expanded market for cholesterol-lowering drugs that will result from even the most careful application of the guidelines on a national scale. The public will benefit from reductions in coronary risk and disease. And government will benefit from better health of its citizens and from reduced national expenditures that should result from reductions in coronary risk and disease. . .

"Moreover, this concordance of interests should promote cooperation—even collaboration—on the part of these various constituencies, something that is indeed occurring in part in quite a gratifying way.

"In closing, I'd like to acknowledge the pleasure I've had in playing an active role in the national cholesterol campaign. It has been a most exciting year—and a great pleasure this evening to be able to share some of my thoughts with friends and colleagues in the cholesterol and cardiovascular communities."

Goodman, DS. Cholesterol Revisited: Molecule, Medicine and Media. *Arteriosclerosis* 9, 430-438, 1989.

had experienced a nonfatal heart attack, as against 11.1 percent, or 212, of the controls, a difference of 1.1 percentage points. As for fatal heart attacks, the figures were 1.7 and 2.3 percent, a difference of 0.6 percentage points, or 12 individuals.

But in the summary of the paper, these unimpressive results were presented in another way, called "relative risk." The lowering of nonfatal coronary heart attacks was said to be 19 percent and of fatal heart attacks 30 percent. These figures were obtained by comparing the absolute numbers in the treatment group with the absolute numbers in the control group while ignoring the total number of men involved. In essence, the researchers threw out the denominator in their fractions and thus were able to make trivial differences seem important.

And this was not the only way in which the LRC figures were manipulated. In order to reach their 30 percent figure, the LRC directors *included* the uncertain cases, those who may or may not have died from a heart attack, and to reach their 19 percent figure, they *excluded* the uncertain cases. If it had been the other way around, the results would have been 24 percent rather than 30, and 15 rather than 19. In other words, they selected data that gave them the results they were seeking.

Even worse, the LRC directors had lowered their own statistical demands. In a preliminary report,[32] written several years before the trial ended, they had stated that to be convincing, they would accept nothing less than the strongest statistical proof of their findings. In this case, it was a statistical level of 0.01, meaning that the trial results would be 99 percent accurate; and to ensure statistical accuracy, the researchers said they would use the very demanding two-tailed t-test.[33]

Thus, the directors of the LRC trial had begun by embracing the highest standards. Then, after the fact, when it was clear that the results of the trial did not measure up to their hopes, they shifted their demand for accuracy from 0.01 to the much less stringent 0.05 and to the easy one-tailed t-test.

In response to critical letters to the *Journal of the American*

Medical Association, the directors simply denied that they had ever declared in writing the high standards that they had originally intended to satisfy. "The term 'significant' was not defined in terms of a particular statistical probability level," they claimed.[34]

Diet-heart supporters look offended if you tell them that of half a million screened men, a mere 12 were rescued from death in the LRC trial. In fact, the number rescued was actually smaller. Fewer in the treatment group died from heart attacks (32 versus 44), but more died by violence or suicide (11 versus 4). If we calculate in the ingenious way used by the LRC leaders and other diet-heart proponents, using relative risk instead of absolute risk, the excess of violent deaths was huge; after all, eleven is 175 percent greater than four.

Hyping the benefits, minimizing the risks

If all men in the US with blood cholesterol as high as in the LRC study received the same treatment and got the same result, two hundred lives would be saved per year, provided that the LRC result was not merely due to chance. However, in a 1990 letter to the editors of *The Atlantic Monthly*, Dr. Daniel Steinberg, chairman of the conference that started the publicly funded National Cholesterol Education Campaign, declared that 100,000 lives could be saved each year. He further claimed that such amazing results had been demonstrated with statistical significance "in a large number of studies."[35]

Just a few months later, Dr. Basil Rifkind, who had been the director of the LRC study, admitted in a medical journal that the scientific trials had not reduced the number of deaths from coronary heart disease, and that "further gains in life expectancy are unlikely in developed countries."[36]

The LRC trial results were so feeble that they may well have been caused by mere chance. And both the drug used in the study, cholestyramine, and the supposedly innocent placebo taken by the control group produced some extremely unpleasant side effects. Sixty-eight percent of the men taking the cholestyramine experienced gastrointestinal side effects during their first year of treatment: gas, heartburn, belching, bloating, abdominal pain, nausea and vomiting. Almost 50 percent suffered from constipation or diarrhea. In the control group, 43 percent experienced similar side effects during the first year, a far higher rate than what could be expected to occur if the placebo were truly ineffective.

The study's report assured readers that the side effects were not serious, and that they could be neutralized by standard clinical means. The authors noted that after seven years the number of these side effects had decreased to only 29 percent, about the same amount as had occurred in the placebo group. Their words suggested that pains in the stomach and the guts had nothing to do with the cholestyramine treatment but were either due to pure imagination or were symptoms that the test individuals would have had anyway.

In controlled drug trials the control group usually receives an ineffective placebo that does not produce side effects. Researchers want to determine whether symptoms considered as side effects may in fact be accidental symptoms—symptoms that appear by chance—unrelated to the treatment. Accidental symptoms may, of course, occur in the controls also. Therefore, the percentage of side effects in the placebo group is subtracted from the percentage of side effects in the treatment group to give the true percentage of side effects from the drug.

But in the LRC study, subjects received a placebo that certainly was not without side effects. Forty-three percent experienced gastrointestinal distress—a much higher number than one would expect with an innocent placebo. Therefore it is not reassuring to read that the side effects from the drug equaled the side effects from the placebo. (To claim that these frequent side effects were accidental means that 43 percent of all adults suffer from gastrointestinal symptoms. Luckily, this is not true.)

Neither is it reassuring to learn that "the side effects were treated by standard clinical means." These words mean that more than half of these previously healthy individuals had to take, in addition to cholestyramine or a placebo, laxatives, antacids or drugs to stop diarrhea or to prevent nausea and vomiting.

A greater number in the treatment group was also admitted to the hospital for operations or procedures involving the nervous system. No diagnoses or more specific information were given, and as the experimenters were unable to come up with an explanation as to the effect of cholestyramine on the nervous system, these side effects were classified as coincidental. The authors did not consider the possibility that cholesterol reduction in and of itself, and not cholestyramine, may have had a detrimental effect on the nervous system.

Few people know about the many side effects that they may get by taking cholestyramine because they are rarely mentioned to the public. Consider, for example, Dr. Daniel Steinberg's claims in the letter he published in *The Atlantic Monthly*: "The drugs in current use for lowering cholesterol levels have remarkably few

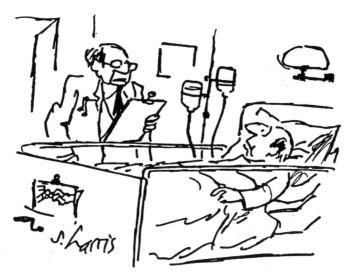

"You'll be glad to know that of the 17 drugs we gave you, and the 43 side effects they caused, we found 6 of the drugs to be effective, and we've cleared up 28 of the side effects."

© 2000 by Sidney Harris

side effects and, to my knowledge, no fatal side effects."[35]

After the LRC trials, diet-heart promoters claimed the following: "Now we have proved that it is worthwhile to lower blood cholesterol; no more trials are necessary. Now it is time for treatment." And they considered treatment necessary for most people.

In the field of clinical science, it is prudent to avoid drawing conclusions about patient groups other than those who have been studied, especially concerning a disease with large age and sex variations. If a treatment is definitely beneficial for middle-aged men with extremely high cholesterol levels, then only middle-aged men with extremely high cholesterol levels should be treated until it has been proven that it is also beneficial for other categories of human beings.

In the LRC it was not even middle-aged men with high cholesterol who were studied but mostly men with inborn errors of cholesterol metabolism. You may recall that it was those with the upper 0.8 percent of the blood cholesterol values who had been selected for the trial. As at least one-half percent of mankind has an inborn error of cholesterol metabolism, then most of the participants must have belonged to that category. Even if we presume that treatment was useful for these individuals, it is not evident that it is also useful for normal individuals.

But the LRC trial directors had no reservations. Not only middle-aged men should be treated but also other age groups, they claimed. And not only men with high blood cholesterol, but also those whose cholesterol was close to normal. And not only men, but also women, even though the LRC trial had not studied women and even though almost all previous studies had shown that high cholesterol is not a risk factor in women, neither is treatment of any use. The only group not included for treatment in the LRC study report was children, an oversight that was corrected later.

No conclusions about dietary intervention can be drawn from the LRC study because both the treatment group and the controls received dietary instruction. The LRC directors admitted as much but that did not deter them from recommending a low-fat, low-cholesterol diet. Instead, they claimed that results from the LRC trial taken together with the large volume of evidence relating diet, plasma cholesterol levels and coronary heart disease, supported the view that cholesterol lowering by diet also would be beneficial.

This argument is typical; no study has proven that animal fat and high cholesterol are dangerous to the heart but if we put all the studies together, they do. In the Alice-in-Wonderland atmosphere of the Lipid Research Clinics, nothing plus nothing conveniently equals something.

Science by citation

The high rate of coronary heart disease in Finland has prompted several researchers in that country to conduct preventive trials; Dr. Tatu Miettinen and his co-workers from Helsinki are among them. (Another, more well-known trial from Helsinki, the Helsinki Heart study, is described on page 176.)

One-half of about 1200 middle-aged, more or less overweight and hypertensive male business executives with high blood cholesterol were advised about smoking, exercise, weight reduction and diet; the other half were used as a control group. If the blood pressure and the blood cholesterol in the treatment group did not become normal, they were also treated with various blood pressure and cholesterol-lowering drugs.

The experimenters were quite satisfied with the effects of their efforts on risk factors. Blood cholesterol fell by 6.3 percent, the blood pressure by about 5 percent. Tobacco consumption fell about 13 percent.

But improved risk factors did not lead to better end results. In the group that exercised, reduced their weight, ate less animal fat and more vegetable oil, and quit smoking, there were twice as many heart attacks as in the control group.[37]

The investigators believed that the greater number of heart attacks in the treatment group was probably due to the use of

drugs—clofibrate, which some had taken to lower their cholesterol, or perhaps to the drugs for high blood pressure. (What a
frightening thought—that drugs which are used on millions of
people to lower their blood pressure or to prevent coronary heart
disease could actually cause the disease instead.)

Their explanation does not jibe with the results of other
studies. In two previous British trials investigators said that clofibrate lowered the number of heart attacks. Other studies have
shown that drugs used against high blood pressure may protect
against coronary heart disease.

The unfavorable result may simply have been due to the
fact that the therapy is ineffective. Therefore, the outcome is determined by chance—in one trial the number of heart attacks is
a little smaller, in another a little greater. But the diet-heart proponents prefer to look only at the supportive studies and ignore
those that are not.

Science Citation Index is an interesting aid for scientists.
Here you can see who has cited any scientific paper, how often it
has been cited and where. Editors of medical journals like to
point out when the papers published in their magazines are frequently cited. Frequent citation indicates influence and is prestigious not only for journals but also for individual scientists. The
names of those who have cited papers by Nobel Prize laureates
take up many columns of small type in *Science Citation Index.*

It is interesting to open the *Index* and see how often the
1985 paper by Miettinen and colleagues has been cited. Let us
compare it with the main report from the LRC trial, published
one year previously. Both papers dealt with the same subject
and were published in the same journal and no one has questioned the honesty of the experimenters or the quality of the studies. It is reasonable to assume that they would be cited almost
equally often. That the LRC trial, at least according to its directors, was supportive, and the Miettinen trial was not, is unimportant because the aim of research is to find the truth, whether
it supports the current theories or not.

Table 6A. Frequency of citation for the Miettinen trial and the LRC trial.

	Miettinen trial	LRC trial
First year	6	109
Second year	5	121
Third year	3	202
Fourth year	1	180

After Ravnskov.[49]

Table 6A shows the frequency with which the two studies were cited during the first four years after their publication. The table shows that scientists are like the rest of us: they forget embarrassing events and recall only pleasant memories. This may be a useful quality when it comes to personal relationships, but it does nothing to further scientific knowledge.

Which do you want: a gastric ulcer or a heart attack?

New cholesterol-lowering drugs require new trials. The previous results were less successful than expected because of side effects of the drugs, said investigators. Their benefits in reducing heart disease were undermined by an increase in deaths due to other reasons, they claimed. Others thought that the drugs had not lowered cholesterol levels sufficiently.

A more recent drug called gemfibrozil (Lopid®) is chemically close to clofibrate, but was considered more favorable because it lowers the total amount of cholesterol in the blood and at the same time increases the "good" cholesterol. This drug was selected for a new trial in Helsinki, Finland, in a project called the Helsinki Heart Study, led by Professor Heikki Frick.[38]

Once again, investigators chose healthy, middle-aged men

with high blood cholesterol. All participants were advised to quit smoking, to exercise and to lose weight. Half of them received gemfibrozil, the others a placebo drug.

As in earlier trials, the number of deaths was equal in the two groups, but for the first time cholesterol lowering resulted in a statistically significant reduction of nonfatal heart attacks. In the Oslo trial, a significant reduction in heart attack deaths was achieved when the participants had combined weight loss and cessation of smoking with cholesterol lowering; in the LRC trial the effect was not significant, according to the usual statistical methods; and in the 1978 WHO trial the smaller number of non-fatal heart attacks was outnumbered by a greater number of fatal ones.

Has science proved that high cholesterol is the killer? May we use the trial of Professor Frick and his colleagues as an argument to institute cholesterol-lowering measures in a large part of the world's population?

According to the diet-heart idea, cholesterol is dangerous because it generates atherosclerosis. If this were true then other vascular diseases caused by atherosclerosis, such as stroke, should also be influenced by a lowering of blood cholesterol. However, in all the trials investigators only used fatal and nonfatal coronary heart disease as end points.

In the tables of all the trials, the reader will find a small group of patients classified as "other cardiovascular diseases." In most trials the number in this category is slightly greater in the treatment group. When the effect of the trial is close to the borderline of statistical significance, as it usually is in the cholesterol trials (except when the effect is not directly negative), the small differences between the numbers of "other cardiovascular diseases" in the treatment and the control groups take on great importance. If all cardiovascular diseases including coronary heart disease are put together in the Helsinki Heart Study, then the result is no longer statistically significant. In other words, the results could easily have been caused by chance.

In addition, the treatment gave unpleasant side effects. During the first year 232 or 11.3 percent of the treated individuals had gastrointestinal symptoms. Gradually the side effects abated. The report did not tell whether the test individuals became accustomed to the drug or whether, as in the LRC trial, they were treated with other drugs to combat the side effects. What we do know is that in the treatment group 81 were operated on for some gastrointestinal ailment. In the control group, only 53 received such operations. Thus, if the difference in the number of heart attacks was real and not caused by chance, the question is this: Would you prefer an operation on your stomach or gall bladder, or a nonfatal heart attack, because the sum of heart attacks and operations was almost identical in the two groups.

The Helsinki trial failed to lower *mortality* from coronary heart disease, and there was no significant difference between the total number of deaths either; if anything, more died in the treatment group than in the control group. But this is not the end of the Helsinki story.

An expedient by-product

Parallel with their study on healthy men, the Finnish researchers performed another experiment on men who had already suffered a heart attack. About 600 such individuals participated, all of whom worked at the same companies as those in the original Helsinki study.[39]

The results after five years were disheartening. Seventeen of those who took gemfibrozil had died from a heart attack compared to only eight in the placebo group.

Dr. Frick and his co-authors were eager to stress that this difference was most probably due to chance. In the summary of the paper they wrote that the number of fatal and nonfatal heart attacks did not differ significantly between the two groups.

They were right, because in contrast to their fellow-directors of the other trials, they used the correct type of statistical analysis for determining the effect of a treatment, the two-tailed

t-test. If they had used the one-sided test as diet-heart supporters usually do to justify allegedly positive effects, the larger number that died in the treatment group would have been statistically significant.

But there are other ways of tweaking the figures. In the group
called "cardiac deaths," the Finnish investigators included a small
group called "unwitnessed deaths," meaning those for whom the
cause of death was unknown. It is not self-evident that an
unwitnessed death is due to a heart attack, and such deaths
should, of course, have been classified otherwise.

In fact, if they had excluded the "unwitnessed deaths," there
were more than *three times* more fatal heart attacks in the treatment group—sixteen versus five. And this difference was indeed
statistically significant.

The directors of the study admitted that the result was not
"in accord with previous experience," but they had a number of
explanations. As the trial was only "an expedient by-product" of
the original trial, the number of individuals had been too small
to give reliable results, they said. They took considerable pains
to explain the low number of heart attacks in the control group.
It was unlikely that it reflected the incidence in the general population, they claimed. Most probably the individuals in the control group had been less affected by coronary atherosclerosis than
those in the treatment group simply because of chance.

Short guts and long lives?

A surgeon at the University of Minnesota Medical School,
Dr. Henry Buchwald, had a bright idea. He had noted that when
the last part of the small intestine is removed from a patient (because of cancer or another disease) his blood cholesterol level
decreases sharply. The explanation is that a great deal of cholesterol and bile acid is taken up in this part of the intestine and, as
cholesterol is used for the production of bile acid in the liver,
considerable amounts of cholesterol are lost in the stool when
the lower part of the small intestine is missing. Could this same

operation be used to treat patients with too much cholesterol in their blood?

In 1963 Dr. Buchwald and his team performed the first ileal bypass to lower cholesterol. The surgeons cut and closed off the last third of the small intestine, and joined the open end of the upper two-thirds to the large intestine. Many such operations have been performed since then, mainly on patients suffering from familial hypercholesterolemia. Unfortunately, only a few researchers have looked at the results of the operation in a controlled study.

Two of them were Dr. Pekka Koivisto and Dr. Tatu Miettinen from Helsinki, Finland.[40] Twenty-seven patients with familial hypercholesterolemia had this operation performed, and after ten years their condition was compared with 27 control patients treated with cholesterol-lowering drugs and matched for a large number of the usual risk factors for coronary disease.

The ileal bypass was indeed effective, more effective than the drugs. The final level of cholesterol was 23 percent lower in the operated patients, and the LDL-cholesterol was even better, at 27 percent lower than in the controls. But there was no difference in the final outcome. After ten years, five of the patients receiving operations and four of the controls had died from a heart attack, and three patients in each group had suffered a nonfatal heart attack.

In spite of this disappointing result, Dr. Miettinen and his colleagues recommended ileal bypass as a treatment against high cholesterol. They saw the operation as a partial success because those who had suffered a heart attack in the bypass group had lowered their cholesterol by only 25 percent while those who hadn't had a heart attack had lowered their cholesterol by 33 percent. Obviously they meant more heart attacks could have been prevented if they had succeeded in bringing cholesterol levels down even more.

But it is difficult to see how the cholesterol level had any importance at all, because in the control group the reduction was about ten percent, both in patients who had suffered a heart attack and in those who had not. Furthermore, cholesterol in controls who hadn't had a heart attack was almost 20 percent higher than in the operated patients who had suffered one. Thus, if anything, the bypass operation had induced heart attacks instead of preventing them.

Dr. Buchwald himself, the inventor of the bypass operation, has conducted the largest trial on ileal bypass. In cooperation with 23 colleagues and 51 advisers, he studied more than 800 middle-aged patients, mostly men, who had suffered at least one heart attack. Half of them were chosen at random to receive an ileal bypass while the other half served as controls.[41]

After ten years, 32 in the surgery group had died from coronary heart disease compared to 44 of the controls. In all, 49 had died in the surgery group, 62 in the control group. These differences were far from statistically significant; they could have been due to chance. But in a subgroup analysis Dr. Buchwald and his 23 co-authors found that if only those who had suffered a less serious heart attack initially were considered, the difference was almost statistically significant. (But among those who had a more serious heart attack initially, more had died in the surgery group.)

There were other bright spots. In the control group there were more nonfatal heart attacks, more episodes of severe angina and many more patients underwent heart bypass surgery. If all these events were taken together, the difference between the two groups was highly significant.

Apparently a success. However, a study like this is, of course, neither single nor double blind. It is necessary to remind you of Professor Cornfield's and Dr. Mitchell's conclusion from their early overview of cholesterol-lowering trials: open trials are successful, blind trials are not. To decide whether a patient has had a heart attack or something else, or whether a patient should have a coronary graft or not, is a highly subjective matter. You would need to be a saint to avoid letting ulterior motives influence your judgment in a million-dollar trial with so much glory and prestige at stake.

The authors argued that the higher number of heart bypass operations in the control group had improved their survival and blunted the trend toward a reduction in mortality in the surgery group. However, new artery grafts may eliminate your angina, but most studies have shown that they do not prolong your life. On the contrary, a net excess of two deaths in the control group could be ascribed to complications of the artery bypass operations, thus further reducing the difference.

Other complications were produced by the ileal bypass itself. Each year 4 percent of those receiving the operation had a kidney stone, a total of about 135 attacks in all; 14 had their gall bladder removed; and 57 had symptoms of bowel obstruction, 15 of whom required an operation. And there was more.

Lack of the ileum results not only in loss of bile acid but when bile acid is lost, the fats transported with the bile are also lost, making the stool frequent and loose. Loss of fat means loss of calories. On average, ileum bypass patients had a weight loss of 5.3 kg, which means that some patients may have lost only a few kilograms but others may have lost up to ten or more.

You may probably recall Dr. Kannel's words about the "formidable risk" of coronary heart disease contributed by obesity. An ileal bypass is an effective treatment against obesity, and obese patients must therefore have been in great excess in the control group. It is difficult to know how many extra heart attacks among controls were due to obesity, but this bias should at least have been mentioned in the discussion and summary of the report.

Can atherosclerosis disappear?

Trials that include thousands of individuals are laborious and, of course, extremely expensive. In recent years scientists have taken a shortcut. Instead of coronary deaths they have used "regression of coronary artery disease" as a measure of treatment effect. By regression they mean a widening, or at least a less rapid narrowing, of the coronary arteries as seen in coronary angiography. An increase in the mean diameter of the coronary vessels during treatment is said to be due to disappearance of atheromas, the scientific name for the vascular deposits or plaques seen in atherosclerosis. Angiographic trials are much cheaper because they can be performed with fewer test individuals and it is also possible to evaluate the results after a much shorter time.

The use of laboratory changes rather than the number of deaths as a measure of treatment effect is called a "surrogate outcome." The term "surrogate" is used because it is not self-evident that laboratory changes can be translated into clinical effects such as lowering of mortality. It is also questionable whether widening of a coronary vessel observed by angiography can be interpreted as the disappearance of an atheroma, a subject we shall explore later on. Let us first have a look at the angiographic trials.

The National Heart, Lung and Blood Institute and the American Heart Association support the diet-heart idea one hundred percent. Most of those who have introduced the cholesterol campaign or have advocated it most vigorously are members, or have previously been members, of the National Heart, Lung, and Blood Institute or the American Heart Association. Together these two groups administer more than 90 percent of all grants for cardiovascular research, which means that researchers critical to the diet-heart idea have little chance of obtaining financial support.

In the early 1980s, the National Heart, Lung and Blood Institute decided to study the effect of cholesterol lowering as measured directly by x-ray angiograms. To lower cholesterol they chose cholestyramine (Atromidin®), the same drug used in the ongoing LRC trial. For five years, researchers studied 116 male patients with coronary heart disease and high blood cholesterol; one-half received cholestyramine, the other half a placebo drug.[42]

The results were again disappointing. In the treatment group the coronary arteries widened a fraction of a millimeter in four patients, but they had also become wider in four of the untreated patients.

Before the trial began the investigators had decided to analyze their results using the so-called one-tailed t-test, which makes it possible to obtain statistical significance with much smaller differences between the two groups. As I mentioned earlier, true scientists do not accept this test in treatment trials. The one-tailed t-test is acceptable if the result can go in one direction only, and treatment trials can certainly go in both directions. The number of deaths may either increase or decrease as we have seen in several cholesterol-lowering trials, but the National Heart, Lung and Blood Institute approved the use of the one-tailed t-test because they believed that "the weight of laboratory and epidemiological evidence" provided assurance that the results could only go in one direction.

If you haven't skipped too many chapters you will probably agree with me that the weight of laboratory and epidemiological evidence suggests nothing of the kind. Let me only mention that when the study they initiated was published in 1984, not fewer than seven controlled cholesterol-lowering trials had resulted in an increase in coronary mortality in the treatment groups compared to controls.

By using the one-tailed t-test and by manipulating the figures in different ways, the 15 directors of the study headed by Dr. John Brensike found a combination that gave statistical support for the benefit of the treatment. Actually, the only finding of interest was a tendency to more atherosclerotic progress in the patients whose HDL-cholesterol (the so-called good guy) went down during the trial and in patients whose LDL-cholesterol (the so-called bad guy) was high from the beginning. They admitted that the result was not exactly what they had expected, but in a later paper[43] they stated that the improvement was proportional with the changes in blood cholesterol they had seen in the patients independent of whether they had been treated or not. In other words, the coronary vessels had not worsened as often if the cholesterol was low rather than high. In fact, such changes were anticiapted because we know that high LDL predicts CHD and therefore atherosclerosis also.

It is easy for cholesterol researchers to get caught up in circular reasoning. We do not yet know the cause of atherosclerosis. What we do know is that high cholesterol is a risk factor. Theoretically, high blood cholesterol may be the cause, but high cholesterol may also be secondary to the real cause; the causative factors may have induced atherosclerosis and at the same time it may have raised the level of cholesterol circulating in the blood. The aim of the study was to determine which of these alternatives was true. If cholesterol is the bad guy, a reduction in its concentration should be followed by a decrease in atherosclerosis, or at least by a halting of its progress. If cholesterol is only an innocent bystander, witnessing the crime and being influenced by it, then a reduction in its concentration would not have any effect because the unknown villain is still at large. Crime is not prevented by killing the witnesses.

"Selective blindness"

With the support of the National Heart, Lung and Blood Institute and Upjohn, Dr. David Blankenhorn and his group from the University of Southern California medical department started a new angiographic trial, called CLAS, the Cholesterol-Lowering Atherosclerosis Study.[44]

This study included 162 patients who had undergone coronary bypass operations. After routine laboratory tests, all major arteries were examined by angiography. The patients were then randomly assigned to two groups of equal size. One group took cholesterol-lowering drugs while the other took ineffective placebo tablets. The study was "blinded," meaning that neither the patients nor the doctors knew which group got treatment and which did not. To be sure that cholesterol was lowered sufficiently, treatment patients received two drugs at the same time—colestipol (Colestid®) and nicotinic acid.

After two years of treatment, another angiography was performed. Researchers found that the arteries had widened in 16 percent of those who had received the drugs compared to only 2 percent of the control patients. In 38 percent of the treated patients the diameter of the vessels had decreased, but this finding was seen as a success because the vessels had narrowed in a higher percentage of the controls, about 56 percent.

And the differences were statistically significant, according to Dr. Blankenhorn and his colleagues, but only because they used the one-tailed t-test.

It may seem petty to take exception to the details of statistical formulas, and if the authors had underlined the weakness of their study and pointed out the questionable results themselves, no further discussion would be necessary. But the authors did not hint at any weakness. Their remarkable deviation from standard statistical practice was not even mentioned in the summary of the paper (often the only part of a paper that is read), nor when Blankenhorn's study was cited in other publications. Furthermore, there was another problem.

The side effects of nicotinic acid, one of the drugs used in the study, are so obvious that no one can have any doubt about who is taking the drug, least of all the patient. Shortly after having swallowed the tablet, the patient feels his skin burning and itching as if stung by nettles. Patients can't help but talk about the side effects to all who will listen, including their doctors.

If the doctors still wanted to know for certain whether the patient had treatment or not, they could look into the laboratory records. To be sure that the cholesterol really went down during the study, patients in the treatment group took the drugs during a period of three months before the start of the trial, and those whose cholesterol did not go down as much as was anticipated were excluded.

And cholesterol went down. On average blood cholesterol decreased by 26 percent in those who took the drugs; the "bad" cholesterol decreased by as much as 43 percent. On their regular visits to their doctors the patients might as well have had a sign around their necks telling whether they belonged to the treatment or to the control group.

Thus, the trial was neither single- nor double-blind, which the authors had the honesty to admit. They called it "selective blind," a new and striking description of that branch of the research tree where the cholesterol hawks are breeding.

A researcher may be utterly impartial and dedicated to the truth, but he is probably not a saint. Human nature is such that when doctors know to which group a patient belongs, their judgment will be influenced in at least some of the cases no matter how much they try to avoid this bias.

But Dr. Blankenhorn's group was so certain of the results that they immediately called a press conference at the National Heart, Lung and Blood Institute and, with much fanfare, announced the sensational findings.[45] Now, at last, "for the first time," they had shown "a strong and consistent therapy effect from cholesterol lowering at the level of coronary arteries."

Dr. Blankenhorn must have forgotten that Dr. Brensike and his co-workers claimed to have proven this several times. As you probably recall, it was Dr. Brensike's "strong laboratory and epidemiological evidence" that allowed Dr. Blankenhorn and his colleagues to make use of the one-tailed t-test.

But Dr. Blankenhorn went further. He also claimed that his studies demonstrated that blood cholesterol should be brought down to a level of 185 mg/dl, guidelines that were soon after adopted as national policy by the National Heart, Lung, and Blood Institute and the American Heart Association.

What an amazing situation! Remember that even the strongest supporters of the diet-heart idea do not believe that diet is sufficient to lower cholesterol as much as in Dr. Blankenhorn's trial; instead drugs must be used. How many adults have cholesterol above the 185 level? According to Dr. Basil Rifkind, one of the strongest advocates for the diet-heart idea, it probably amounts to 40 million healthy Americans. Said Robert Levy, former head of the American Heart Association, the results were "exciting," even if they were not quite unexpected. And the directors of the Upjohn Company, producers of colestipol, must have been delighted.

In a scientific report, it is customary to include discussion of the results of other investigators, especially when they deviate completely from one's own results. How did Dr. Blankenhorn and his co-workers, and the brain trust at the National Heart, Lung and Blood Institute, comment on the disheartening results of Drs. Bemis, Kimbiris, Shub, Kramer and their groups (see pages 130-131), who didn't find the slightest connection between changes in cholesterol levels in the coronary vessels and changes in cholesterol levels in the blood? How did they explain the fact that the coronary vessels improved in their own experiments, but not in the many previous studies where cholesterol went down just as much or more? Why did they place more importance on their own dubiously positive results than on the many indisputable negative ones? I cannot give you an answer because they did not comment on them at all.

Something better

Three years later, in 1990, the results from a new angiographic trial were published by Dr. Greg Brown and his team in Washington, DC, again supported by the National Heart, Lung and Blood Institute.[46] Obviously the "strong and consistent" effect of Blankenhorn's treatment was not enough to make further studies unnecessary. In their paper they wrote that the lipid changes in the previous trials—including Dr. Blankenhorn's—were small and the clinical benefits limited. Dr. Brown and his colleagues also used two drugs at the same time. Thirty-eight men received colestipol (Colestid®) along with lovastatin, one of the new and more effective cholesterol-lowering drugs (see later); 36 received nicotinic acid and colestipol; and 46 received a placebo. The trial was designed as a double-blind study. Most of the men participating had familial hypercholesterolemia.

And indeed their cholesterol levels came down; by 34 percent in the lovastatin-colestipol group and by 23 percent in the niacin-colestipol group. The devil himself, LDL-cholesterol, was lowered even more, by 45 percent and 32 percent, respectively.

Before and after treatment the width of the coronary arteries was measured at various points using a fivefold magnification of the x-ray pictures. Magnification was necessary because, on average, the vessel diameters in the niacin-colestipol group increased by a mere 0.04 mm only, whereas the diameters in the lovastatin-colestipol decreased by 0.002 mm and in the control group by 0.05 mm. These were small differences, indeed, but they were statistically significant, and Dr. Brown and his colleagues saw them as a proof of therapeutical success.

I am sure you noticed that the vessel diameters *decreased* in those treated with lovastatin-colestipol, the ones who had their cholesterol lowered the most. In some parts of the arteries the diameter had actually increased, but on average, taking all measurements together, the diameters had decreased. A decrease of the diameters means, of course, that the coronary vessels had become narrower, which is certainly not an improvement, although the diameter in the control group decreased even more. The authors offered no comment about this striking finding, nor about the fact that the only two deaths in the study—and the only heart attack—were seen in the lovastatin-colestipol group. In fact, the title of their paper said the opposite: "Regression [meaning 'improvement"] of coronary artery disease as a result of intensive lipid-lowering therapy. . . "

The anguish of angiography

Let us keep in mind that a change in diameter of the coronary artery is nothing but a surrogate outcome. It is assumed that a widening of a coronary vessel on an x-ray means less atherosclerosis and thus a better chance to avoid a heart attack, but this is only an assumption.

Artery walls are surrounded by smooth muscle cells. When such cells contract, the artery narrows. When they relax, it widens. Various factors may stimulate the smooth muscle cells of the coronary arteries to contract including mental stress, anxiety, exposure to cold and even a sustained hand grip. The latter effect was studied six years earlier by Dr. Greg Brown, the same Dr. Brown who led the angiographic trial mentioned above. He found that a hand grip sustained for a few minutes was followed by a 35 percent decrease in the vessel diameter.[47]

Consider that the changes seen in the trials were only a few percent on average. What would your reaction be if somebody were to put a long catheter all the way from your groin up to your heart and into your coronary vessels? If you are not a stuntman or an astronaut, you probably would have gripped the nurse's hand or something else very tightly, at least during the first examination. How, then, did the researchers know whether an increase in blood vessel diameter at the second examination was due to the patient being more relaxed or to the vessels being less atherosclerotic?

The study outcome may also have been influenced by the fact that almost all coronary patients receive drugs that relax the coronary vessels. In the trial, Dr. Brown and his co-workers were aware of that problem. The use of such drugs was "duplicated as exactly as possible." This can't have been too easy because the level of any drug in the blood depends on a large number of factors that are difficult to standardize. And Dr. Brown and his colleagues didn't write anything about duplicating possible hand grips or anxious feelings because such duplication is, of course, impossible. So, any factor that may influence the state of the smooth muscle cells in the coronary vessels may have influenced the vessel diameter far more than the possible appearance or disappearance of a tiny amount of cholesterol.

There are more uncertainties. Dr. Seymor Glagov and his colleagues from University of Chicago studied the hearts of 136 deceased individuals and found that when vessels become sclerotic, they actually widen to compensate for the narrowing brought about by the deposition of cholesterol in their walls. In fact, this widening overcompensates for the deposition until the cholesterol deposits occupy about 40 percent of the area beneath the muscle wall.[48] Only thereafter does the vessel become steadily narrower. In other words, an increase of vessel diameter may be due to better relaxation of the vessel wall or disappearance of cholesterol in a highly sclerotic vessel, but it also could be due to a compensatory widening during the first stages of cholesterol deposition. How could the trial directors know which of these alternatives explained the increase in vessel diameter?

Meta-analysis

Certain treatments are easy to assess. The right antibiotic, for instance, will cure nine out of ten women with an uncomplicated urinary infection, which means that after having treated fewer than a dozen patients and controls for a few days you already know for certain that the drug is effective. But after the many cholesterol-lowering trials, scientists still don't know whether the treatment could change mortality. Statisticians say that to prove a beneficial effect on mortality, many more test individuals are necessary, probably more than 100,000. (If the beneficial effect of treatment is so difficult to prove, aren't we justified in concluding that high cholesterol cannot be that dangerous for our health?)

But the problem may be solved in another way. The solution is called meta-analysis.

In a meta-analysis, data from all studies that satisfy certain standards of quality are put together in the hope that they will provide a large enough sample for statistical reliability. For medical trials, at least, three standards are mandatory. Trials should be double-blind, they should be controlled, and the test individuals and the controls should be chosen randomly. Also, in order to use the accumulated results from many trials, it is necessary for the same kind of treatment to have been used in each trial and, of course, the result of the treatment—the outcome or the end point—should also be the same.

By now you may have realized that if all standards are to be satisfied, very few trials can qualify. Very few trials have been performed in a true double-blind fashion, and besides cholesterol-lowering, some trials have also used other kinds of intervention. Nevertheless, let us have a look at the entire body of trials that have been published before 1994, the year of the first statin trial.

Several meta-analyses on cholesterol-lowering trials have been published. When I prepared the first edition of this book in Swedish, it annoyed me that most of these analyses had excluded a number of trials, particularly the unsupportive ones. So I decided to perform a meta-analysis myself that included *all* randomized and controlled trials where the aim had been to lower cholesterol, whether by diet or by drugs, and whether or not they had also used other kinds of intervention.[49] I included open trials, since it was not possible to do a fair selection of double-blind studies because even trials that were designated as double-blind studies were, in fact, more or less open for the reasons I have given above. The raw figures for my meta-analysis are given in Table 6B.

As you can see, the number of deaths from a heart attack was equal in the treatment and in the control groups, and the *total* number of deaths was greater in the treatment groups. In one study total mortality had decreased significantly, in two others it had increased significantly, and in no trial was coronary mortality changed more than could be attributed to chance. More sophisticated calculations did not change the picture.

There was a small reduction in the number of nonfatal heart attacks. Calculated as a reduction in "relative risk," the way diet-heart supporters usually do, the difference was 9.7 percent; calculated in the appropriate way as a reduction in rate or "absolute risk," the difference was 0.3 percent. Due to the large number of individuals studied, this small difference was

Table 6B. Overall results of 26 controlled cholesterol-lowering trials. The number of individuals in the three calculations is not identical because a few trials did not give the number for all end points.

	Treatment Groups	Control Groups
Number of individuals	59,514	53,251
Nonfatal heart attacks	2.8%	3.1%
Number of individuals	60,824	54,403
Fatal heart attacks	2.9%	2.9%
Number of individuals	60,456	53,958
Total number of deaths	6.1%	5.8%

After Ravnskov.[49]

statistically significant, but most probably it was the result of bias because most of the trials were open and some of them were multifactorial.

But another finding definitely proved that cholesterol lowering does not provide any benefit. If cholesterol lowering could reduce the risk of coronary heart disease, a pronounced and prolonged decline in cholesterol values should, of course, lower the risk more than a slight and short one. But there was no relationship between the degree of cholesterol reduction and any of the end points, not between individuals in each trial and not between trials. And, on average, total mortality was equal in short and long trials, and coronary mortality was *higher* in long trials than in short ones.

So, although some of the trials also included physical exercise, weight loss, reduction of blood pressure and smoking advice, and although most trials were open, the number of avoided nonfatal heart attacks was not larger than 0.3 percent. And even if knowledge about their patients' group affiliation had not influenced the participating doctors, remember from Chapter 1 that what doctors—even experienced ones—call a heart attack is often something else.

After its publication in the *British Medical Journal*, my meta-analysis provoked harsh comments from diet-heart supporters.[50] According to my critics, the most serious mistake was to include trials using female sex hormones, since such drugs are now considered toxic to the heart. (Three unsuccessful trials used estrogen treatment.) But in one of the first controlled trials published, conducted by Professor Jeremiah Stamler, the researchers used low doses of the female sex hormone estrogen, and that trial had the best result of all.[51] High doses of estrogen are possibly harmful for men, but whether low doses are harmful is an open question. In women, at least, low doses, such as those used in postmenopausal hormone replacement therapy, seemed to protect against heart attacks.[52] The results were also just as unsupportive in the subgroup calculations, even in subgroups that did not include the hormone trials.

Another objection was that I had ignored the angiographic trials, because they "can lead to regression of atheroma," as one of the critics noted. But inclusion of the few angiographic trials that had been published at that time would not have changed the overall result of the meta-analysis either because of their small size. However, let us look at a more recent meta-analysis that did include the angiographic trials.

In this analysis, Dr. George Davey Smith at the Department of Public Health, University of Glasgow, Scotland, and his co-workers excluded the multifactorial trials to study the effect of cholesterol lowering only, and they limited their analysis to total mortality.[53] They ranged the trials in order of risk according to the coronary mortality in the control groups. In high-risk trials, many control individuals died from a heart attack; in low-risk trials relatively few.

Trials in which the control group had the highest mortality were classified as high-risk trials. In this group (which included 5115 individuals in ten trials on the uppermost part of the risk list), mortality had decreased. In the median-risk group (which included 24,090 subjects in 15 trials), mortality was unchanged. In the low-risk group (which was the largest and included 27,918 subjects in ten trials on the lowermost part of the list), mortality had increased. Both the decrease and the increase of total mortality was statistically significant. Overall, in trials where drugs had been used to lower cholesterol, mortality from non-coronary causes had increased significantly. The authors' conclusion was that benefits from cholesterol-lowering drugs seem to be produced only in a small proportion of patients at very high risk of death from coronary heart disease. Thus, in the future, cholesterol lowering should include only individuals at very high risk. But herein lies a problem.

Individuals in the so-called low-risk group were only at low risk compared with individuals in the other two groups. In comparison with normal individuals, they were at high risk also. For instance, their cholesterol was 278 mg/dl on average, higher than in the other two groups. Remember that the lower limit for drug treatment, according to the 1987 recommendations of the National Heart, Lung and Blood Institute, was 185 mg/dl; according to the cholesterol campaign it is 240 mg/dl. Furthermore, half of the trials in the so-called low-risk group were of the secondary preventive type, which means that they included patients who had already suffered a heart attack. Such patients have always been considered as being at high risk. Many of the individuals in the low-risk group were exposed to other risk factors also, so indeed this group was actually a sample of high-risk individuals. How can we discriminate between these high-risk individuals and the high-risk individuals who are said to benefit from cholesterol lowering? The simple fact is that we can't. Even doctors who treat only high-risk individuals may end up shortening the lives of their patients instead of prolonging them, at least if they prescribe the drugs used in these trials.

It is also questionable whether mortality really was lowered in the high-risk trial group. One of the trials, for example, was a multifactorial trial that had been included by mistake. The good result in that trial could therefore have been caused by something other than cholesterol lowering. The other trials were very small, and in only one of these was mortality lowered significantly. There was only one reasonably large trial in the high-risk group, but in that trial mortality had increased.

Anyone who has read scientific papers or official recommendations about cholesterol and the heart knows that the official story is quite different from the one I have described. Listen, for instance, to the recommendations of the European Atherosclerosis Society, published before the advent of the statin drugs: "Clinical trials of secondary prevention by lowering plasma cholesterol, when studied together by meta-analysis, show that morbidity and mortality from coronary disease are reduced; there is also a trend to lower total mortality."[54]

This misleading statement is not unique; in fact, it is typical of diet-heart writings. Similar statements were published in numerous scientific papers in the mass media. You have most likely read such passages yourself.

There is more than one explanation for the inappropriately optimistic messages that doctors and scientists write in support of the diet-heart idea. Their main technique is to cite only the supportive trials. On average, I found that trials considered supportive by their directors had been cited almost six times more often than unsupportive trials. The fact that a trial was cited frequently had little to do with its quality, or whether it had been published in a famous or a less well-known journal. The trial directors themselves had been especially unwilling to cite an unsupportive trial; between 1970 and 1992, no trial considered unsupportive by their directors had been cited in any other trial report. Even authors of meta-analyses selected trials according to their outcome.

Thus far, I have described the many previous, unsuccessful cholesterol-lowering trials. Now let us consider the successful ones. But if you think that here, finally, comes the evidence for the importance of blood cholesterol, you are wrong, because the striking finding in these trials was that although the risk of cardiovascular disease was lowered, it is evident that it must have been due to something other than cholesterol reduction.

A successful dietary trial

The idea that a Mediterranean diet—whatever that is—would be beneficial for cardiovascular disease inspired the French researcher Dr. Michel de Lorgeril and his co-workers from various institutions and hospitals in Lyon, France, to start a new dietary trial, the Lyon Diet-Heart study.[55] About 600 patients who had survived a heart attack were included. Half of the patients were instructed to adopt the so-called Mediterranean diet by including more bread, more root and green vegetables and more fish, and by reducing consumption of red meat (beef and lamb). Participants were instructed to eat fruit every day, to replace pork with poultry and to replace butter and cream with margarine—which was supplied free for the whole family. The margarine used was made with rapeseed (canola) oil, which has a high content of α-linolenic acid, a polyunsaturated fatty acid.

Control group individuals also got dietary advice; they were recommended the usual "prudent" diet, but, except for the margarine, it is not clear from the study report in which way this diet deviated from the experimental diet.

The researchers chose to study α-linolenic acid because of a study by Dr. G. W. Sandker and co-workers from the Department of Human Nutrition at the Agricultural University in Wageningen, the Netherlands.[56] They found that people from Crete, the Greek island where heart attacks were rare (see Chapter 2), had three times more of this fatty acid in their blood than the people from Zutphen, the Netherlands, another district in the Seven Countries study. The Lyon researchers therefore thought that α-linolenic acid might be protective because the rate of heart attacks was much higher in Zutphen than on Crete although their cholesterol levels were almost identical.

(What the Dutch researchers really should have done was to analyze the blood of the people from Corfu, the Greek island where heart attacks were 12 times higher than on Crete. As you probably remember, not only did these people have cholesterol levels similar to those of the inhabitants on Crete, but all other risk factors were also similar. If the only difference between these two populations had been the level of α-linolenic acid in the blood or in the fat tissue, then we would have had a strong argument for a protective effect of this fatty acid. But lots of risk factors were different between the inhabitants on Crete and the people of Zutphen, so why zero in on just one, α-linolenic acid?)

After just six months, a significant difference was found; in the control group 20 individuals had died, compared to only eight in the treatment group.[55] After four years the trial was ended because the improvement in the treatment group had continued; 24 had died in the control group but only 14 in the treatment group. The difference in nonfatal heart attacks was even larger—25 in the control group, but only eight in the treatment group—and it was therefore considered unethical to continue the trial.[57]

For the first time a dietary trial had succeeded in lowering the risk of dying from a heart attack. But which of the ingredients had helped? The authors suggested that it was α-linolenic acid, but other studies give conflicting results. In support is a study by Professor A. Ascherio and his co-workers from Harvard School of Public Health.[58] They asked more than 40,000 healthy health professionals about their diet. Ten years later they found that those who developed coronary heart disease had consumed slightly less α-linolenic acid than those who had had remained free of CHD.

A more reliable method to study how much of a certain fatty acid has been eaten is to study its level in the blood or, even better, in the adipose (fat) tissue. The first method was used by

Dr. G. C. Leng and his team at the Department of Public Health Sciences in Edinburgh, Scotland. They measured α-linolenic acid in the blood of about 1100 individuals, and could not find any difference between individuals with and without CHD.[59] The other method was used in a meticulous study performed by research groups from various university institutions in nine countries under the guidance of Professor Eliseo Gualla at the Department of Epidemiology and Biostatistics, the National School of Health in Madrid.[60] They analyzed the content of α-linolenic acid in fat tissue samples from 639 patients with CHD and 700 control individuals. This method is more reliable because the content of a fatty acid in the tissue reflects the intake over a longer period of time, not just the past 24 hours (as in most dietary studies) or the past few days (as in studies on the levels in the blood). Again, no difference was found between patients with heart disease and control individuals.

Thus, although the Lyon trial seems promising, we don't know why. It could hardly have been the additional α-linolenic acid because other studies indicate that this fatty acid is not protective. But could it have been the extra fruit or vegetables? Or the extra bread? Or the extra fish or chicken?

Or could the apparent benefit have been due to the fact that this trial was a relatively small one? Although the well-known risk factors were evenly distributed in both groups, we do not know all risk factors, and in small trials we cannot be sure that unknown risk factors are represented evenly in the two groups. It seems wise, therefore, to await a confirmation of these results from other research groups before we herald the so-called Mediterranean diet as the final solution. (But don't deprive yourselves of French, Greek or Italian food—it can be very good!)

We can be confident that the benefit achieved in the Lyon trial was not due to a lowering of cholesterol because in both groups the "bad" cholesterol decreased and the "good" cholesterol increased in equal amounts! This surprising finding (at least it may appear surprising to those who have not read this book), that the therapeutical benefit was independent of the degree of cholesterol lowering, we shall meet again in the trials of the statins, a new family of cholesterol-lowering drugs.

Statins: The new wonder drugs

In the late 1980s, the pharmaceutical companies introduced a new type of cholesterol-lowering drug called the "statins." These drugs inhibit the body's production of many important substances, one of which is cholesterol.

Sold as Zocord®, Mevacor®, Pravachol®, Lescol® and Lipitor®, these new drugs have received wide acclaim because of their supposed lack of serious side effects and, in particular, because of the substantial cholesterol reduction they can achieve. Whereas the earlier drugs could lower cholesterol by 15-20 percent at most, the statins can lower cholesterol by 30-40 percent or more. Consequently, large clinical and angiographic trials have ensued. As of January 2000, the results from five large, controlled, randomized and double-blind studies, including more than 30,000 test individuals, and numerous angiographic trials have been published. More data will come.

The results of the five clinical trials, as well as from one yet-to-be published, the EXCEL study, are summarized in Table 6C (pages 202-203).

4S—The Scandinavian Simvastatin Survival Study

In 1994 the results from a large Scandinavian, multicenter trial using simvastatin (Zocord®) were published.[61] The results were noteworthy, indeed. For the first time a trial had succeeded in significantly lowering the risk of both fatal and nonfatal coronary heart disease, and even total mortality. The results were heralded in a famous medical journal: "Lower patients' cholesterol now! There is no longer any doubt about the benefit and safety of treating hypercholesterolemia in patients who have had a myocardial infarction."[62]

The results of the 4S trial were published in *The Lancet* on

November 19 and presented on the same day at a press conference arranged by the producer of simvastatin, Merck Sharp & Dohme. At the conference, Noble Prize winner Joseph Goldstein (see page 95) proclaimed: "This is Christmas Eve!" In the vigorous marketing that followed, simvastatin was heralded as "the missing link."

The study was performed in cooperation with 94 Scandinavian medical departments and directed by Dr. Terje Pedersen from the cardiology section at Aker Hospital, Norway. The steering committee and monitoring staff also included employees from Merck Sharp & Dohme, the sponsor of the trial and the manufacturer of the drug that was tested in the study.

Altogether 4444 men and women with a previous heart attack were treated, half with simvastatin, half with a placebo. After 5.4 years, 8.5 percent had died from a heart attack in the control group, compared with 5 percent in the treatment group. (See Table 6C.) This improvement included men only; the number of women who had died from a heart attack was equal in both groups.

But there were other benefits. The number of nonfatal heart attacks had been lowered even more, from 22.6 percent in the control group to 15.9 percent in the simvastatin group, a gain of 6.7 percent. Furthermore, the number of strokes was reduced significantly, from 4.3 percent to 2.7 percent.

CARE, the Cholesterol and Recurrent Events Trial
A similar study, the CARE trial, conducted by Dr. Franck Sacks and his co-workers from seven American, Canadian and British university hospitals, used pravastatin (Pravachol®) to lower cholesterol, again in patients with a previous heart attack.[63] After five years, 5.7 percent had died from CHD in the control group, compared to only 4.6 percent in the treatment group. Considering the large number of participants, this result doesn't seem particularly impressive and, indeed, it was not statistically significant. In fact, the reduction in CHD deaths was offset by the

Table 6C. Statin Drug Studies

	EXCEL[76]	4S[61]
Trial (after 1 year)		
Drug	Lovastatin	Simvastatin
Length of trial in years	?	5.4
Type of participants	Healthy people with high cholesterol	CHD patients with high cholesterol
Number of participants in drug/control group	6600/1650	2221/2223
Percent male	59	82
Age	18-70	35-70
Cholesterol at start		
LDL-cholesterol, mean	180	190
LDL-cholesterol, range	--	--
Total cholesterol, mean	258	263
Total cholesterol, range	--	215-312
Degree of lowering:		
LDL-cholesterol	?	35%
Total cholesterol	?	25%
Total number of deaths		
Drug/control group, absolute numbers	?	182/256
Drug/control group, percent	0.5/.02	8.2/11.5
Relative risk reduction, percent	+150	-29
Absolute risk reduction, percent	+0.3	-3.3
Statistical significance	?	***
Number of CHD deaths:		
Drug/control group, absolute numbers	?	111/189
Drug/control group, percent	?	5/8.5
Relative risk reduction, percent	?	-41
Absolute risk reduction, percent	?	-3.5
Statistical significance	?	***
Numbers of non-fatal CHD:		
Drug/control group, absolute numbers	?	353/502
Drug/control group, percent	?	15.9/22.6
Relative risk reduction, percent	?	-30
Absolute risk reduction, percent	?	-6.7
Statistical significance	?	***
Similar effects in both sexes	?	no
Effect on all age groups	?	yes
Effect on other cardiovascular diseases	?	yes
Effect independent of degree of cholesterol lowering	?	yes[68]

Statistical Significance: NS means not statistically significant. This result is therefore most likely, but not necessarily, due to chance.
* means that the result may be due to chance in 5 percent of such studies

Table 6C: Statin Drug Studies

WOSCOPS[64]	CARE[63]	AFCAPS/TexCAPS[65]	LIPID[66]
Pravastatin	Pravastatin	Lovastatin	Pravastatin
4.4	5	5.2	6.1
Healthy people with high cholesterol	CHD patients with normal cholesterol	Healthy people with normal cholesterol	CHD patients with all levels
3302/3293	2081/2078	3304/3301	4512/4502
100	86	85	83
45-64	21-75	men 45-73	31-75
		women 55-73	
192	139	150	150
>155	115-174	131-191	--
272	209	221	218
>252	<240	181-266	155-271
26	28	26	25
20	20	19	18
106/135	180/196	80/77	498/633
3.2/4.1	8.6/9.4	2.4/2.3	11/14.1
-21	-8	+3.9	-21
-0.9	-0.77	+0.09	-3
NS	NS	NS	***
38/52	96/119	11/15	287/373
1.2/1.6	4.6/5.7	0.33/0.45	6.4/8.3
-27	-19	-27	-23
-0.42	-1.1	-0.12	-1.9
NS	NS	NS	***
143/204	135/173	116/183[a]	336/463
4.3/6.2	6.5/8.3	3.5/5.5	7.4/10.3
-22	-22	-38	-27
-1.8	-1.8	-2	-2.9
***	*	***	***
--	yes	yes	yes
yes	yes	yes	yes
no	yes	--	yes
yes	yes	yes	Not studied

** means that the result may be due to chance in 1% of such studies
*** means that the result may be due to chance in 0.1% of such studies
a included severe angina

fact that in the treatment group a few more had died from other causes.

There were other benefits, however. As in the 4S trial, the number of strokes was smaller in the treatment group, 2.6 percent compared to 3.8 percent in the control group, and there were also fewer nonfatal heart attacks, 6.4 percent versus 8.3 percent. This effect was most pronounced for women.

WOSCOPS,
the West of Scotland Coronary Prevention Study

The two statin trials mentioned above studied the effect on patients who already had CHD. Is it possible as well to prevent heart disease in healthy individuals whose only "abnormality" is high cholesterol? This was the question asked by Professor James Shepherd and his co-workers from various institutions and hospitals associated with the University of Glasgow, Scotland.[64] To that end they assigned more than 6000 middle-aged men with average cholesterol levels of 272 to receive either pravastatin (Pravachol®) or a placebo drug. Five years later 1.6 percent of the men had died from CHD in the control group against 1.2 percent in the pravastatin group. This difference was far from statistically significant, but in the treatment group fewer had also died from stroke and various noncardiovascular diseases. If deaths from any cause were tabulated, 9.4 percent had died in the control group and 8.6 percent in the pravastatin group, a difference that was close to statistical significance. And the difference between the amount of nonfatal CHD was larger, 6.2 percent versus 4.3 percent.

AFCAPS/TexCAPS, the Air Force/
Texas Coronary Atherosclerosis Prevention Study

Is it possible to prevent heart attacks in healthy individuals with normal cholesterol? If so, it would mean that everyone would benefit from taking a statin drug, starting at middle age and continuing for the rest of their lives. The economical ramifications

are breathtaking, both for the stockholders of the drug companies and, in a less pleasant way, for the directors of health care
systems all over the world who would pay the bill.

A new statin trial was organized to answer the question. It
was directed by the former president of the American Heart Association, Professor Antonio Gotto from Cornell University, New
York, and his co-workers from various institutions and hospitals in Texas. Three of the co-workers were employees at Merck
& Co., the company whose drug lovastatin (Mevacor®) was to be
tested. More than 5000 healthy men and almost 1000 healthy
women with no signs or symptoms of cardiovascular disease were
assigned to treatment, as usual half with the drug, half with a
placebo.

After 5.2 years, 2.3 percent had died in the control group,
versus 2.4 percent in the treatment group. The primary target in
this trial was not the total number of deaths, however, but the
number of fatal and nonfatal heart attacks together with the
amount of severe angina. The difference in combined "events"
was statistically significant, 5.5 percent in the control group versus 3.5 percent in the lovastatin group.[65]

LIPID, another pravastatin trial

The most recent statin trial, cleverly named The Long-term
Intervention with Pravastatin in Ischemic Disease study, or LIPID,
included patients with previous CHD with all ranges of cholesterol levels. This is a logical approach because if the statins prevent cardiovascular disease whether the cholesterol is high or
low, there is no reason to look at people's cholesterol level at all.

This trial was conducted by Drs. Andrew Tonkin and John
Simes at the National Health and Medical Research Council Clinical Trials Center, University of Sydney, Australia, along with a
team of 63 other researchers. Three of the co-workers came from
the drug company Bristol-Myers Squibb.

After six years, total mortality was lowered significantly—by
11 percent in the control group compared to 14 percent in the

treatment group. CHD mortality was lowered by 6.2 percent in the control group and by 8.3 percent in the treatment group. These effects were most pronounced in men. In fact, the benefit for women was much lower and not statistically significant. Again, an effect was seen regardless of the initial total or LDL-cholesterol level, but the effect in patients with LDL-cholesterol below 135 was not statistically significant.[66]

Summing up

In their reports, the directors of these trials cited LDL-cholesterol as an important risk factor in coronary heart disease. But what these trials actually provide, in spite of the glowing reports they received in the press, is strong evidence that cholesterol levels do not matter.

First, the statins were almost as effective for women as they were for men. Indeed, in the CARE trial the effect was most pronounced for the female sex, although almost all studies have shown that high cholesterol is not a risk factor for women.

Second, the elderly were protected just as much as younger individuals, although all studies have shown that high cholesterol is only a weak risk factor, if any at all, for men older than fifty.

Third, the number of strokes was reduced after statin treatment, although all studies have shown that high cholesterol is a weak risk factor for stroke, if at all.

Fourth, patients who had suffered a heart attack were protected even though most studies have shown that high cholesterol is a weak risk factor, if any at all, for those who have already had a heart attack.[67]

Furthermore, the statins protected against coronary heart disease whether the patients' cholesterol was high or low, even though most studies have shown that normal or low cholesterol is not a risk factor for coronary disease.

Most important, there was no association between the degree of cholesterol lowering and the outcome.[68] The risk of having a heart attack was reduced by the same degree whether the cholesterol level was lowered by a large or small amount. As mentioned above, this phenomenon is called "lack of exposure-response." Lack of exposure-response strongly indicates that the factor under investigation is not the true cause, but is secondary to the real cause.

How come the statins are effective for individuals for whom cholesterol is not a risk factor? And how come the effect of the statins does not depend on how much they lower blood cholesterol? If the cholesterol level for these people is not a risk factor for coronary disease, how could a lowering of that cholesterol improve their chances of avoiding a heart attack? If the level of our blood cholesterol is so important, as we have been told for many years, why doesn't it matter whether we lower it by large or small amounts?

The only reasonable explanation is that the statins do more than just lower cholesterol. There is strong evidence for that.[69]

The statins inhibit the body's production of a substance called mevalonate, which is a precursor to cholesterol. When the production of mevalonate goes down, less cholesterol is produced by the cells, and blood cholesterol goes down as well.

But mevalonate is a precursor of other substances as well, substances with important biologic functions.[70] While the metabolic pathways are not known in all details, reduced amounts of mevalonate may explain why simvastatin makes smooth muscle cells less active[71] and platelets less inclined to produce thromboxane.[72] One of the first steps in the process of atherosclerosis is the growth and migration of smooth muscle cells inside the artery walls, and thromboxane is a substance that is necessary for blood clotting. By blocking the function of smooth muscle cells and platelets, simvastatin may benefit cardiovascular disease by at least two mechanisms, both of which are independent of cholesterol levels. Thus, in one of the experiments performed by Japanese researcher Dr. Yusuke Hidaka and his team, the inhibitory effect on the muscle cells could not be abolished by adding LDL-cholesterol to the test tubes;[71] and in experiments that compared the statins with several different cholesterol-lowering agents, thromboxane production was inhibited only by the statins, indicating that the effect was not due to cholesterol reduction itself but to something else.[72]

The protective effects of simvastatin were also demonstrated in animal experiments. In one of them, performed by Dr. B. M. Meiser and colleagues from Munich, Germany, hearts were transplanted into rats.[73] Normally, the function of such grafts gradually deteriorates because the coronary vessels are narrowed by an increased growth of smooth muscle cells in the vascular walls. This condition is called graft vessel disease, a condition with many similarities to early atherosclerosis. In Dr. Meiser's experiment, however, rats that received simvastatin had considerably less graft vessel disease than control rats that did not receive simvastatin, and this was not due to cholesterol reduction as simvastatin does not lower cholesterol in rats. In fact, LDL-cholesterol was highest in the rats that received simvastatin.

In another experiment, Dr. Maurizio Soma and his colleagues from Milan, Italy, placed a flexible collar around one of the carotid arteries in rabbits.[74] After two weeks the arteries with collars became narrow but less so if the rabbits had received simvastatin. Again, the effect had no relation to the rabbits' cholesterol levels.

Thus, the statins in some way protect against cardiovascular disease, but their effect is not due to cholesterol reduction. The proponents of the cholesterol hypothesis have simply had incredible luck in finding a substance that prevents cardiovascular disease and at the same time lowers cholesterol.

But why bother about pharmacological mechanisms? Isn't it wonderful that the statins work? Shouldn't we all take statins?

The costs

To answer that question it is necessary to look at the figures from the trials. To be brief, I have chosen only the figures for coronary death. Take a look at the figures for "number of CHD deaths, relative risk reduction," in Table 6C on pages 202-203. You will find that coronary mortality in these trials was lowered between 19 percent and 41 percent, most in the 4S trial and least in the CARE trial. These are the so-called relative risk figures that are used by most doctors and by the drug companies in their ads. But let us also look at the absolute figures, the "absolute risk reduction," on the next line. Here you will find that death from a heart attack was prevented in only a small percentage of the treated individuals. This figure was highest in the trials that included patients with CHD, whereas it was a trivial 0.12 percent in the AFCAPS/TexCAPS trial, which included healthy individuals with normal cholesterol.

Put another way, the chance of not dying from a heart attack over four to six years for a patient with CHD and high cholesterol is about 92 percent without treatment, and increases to 95 percent with statin treatment.

For healthy individuals, the figures are even less impressive. In the WOSCOPS trial, for instance, the chance of not dying from a heart attack during the five years of the study was 98.4 percent without treatment and 98.8 with treatment. In the AFCAPS/TexCAPS trial, the chance of surviving was 99.55 percent without treatment and 99.67 with treatment.

Let us compare these figures with another kind of treatment, for instance, treatment of urinary tract infections. Nine out of ten patients with a urinary tract infection will recover immediately if treated with an antibiotic for a few days, at the cost of a few dollars for each treatment. But in the 4S trial, for instance, you had to treat 28 patients for five years to prevent one fatal heart attack. So, while one of the patients benefited from the treatment, the others took the drug in vain because they would have survived anyway.

The costs for the drug alone amount to about $150,000 per saved life. In the trials, all expenses are paid by the drug companies, but in real life the patient or society must pay, not only for the costs of the drug but also for the doctors' fees, laboratory analyses and loss of income during the doctor visits. And to prevent one fatal heart attack in healthy people, 235 individuals with high cholesterol and 826 individuals with normal cholesterol have to consume a statin drug for four to five years.

Of course, there may be other gains. Not only did statin treatment prevent coronary death, it also prevented more than twice as many nonfatal heart attacks. We should also subtract the costs for hospital care and other treatments for the patients whose heart attacks we prevent, not to mention the grief and pain associated with the loss of wives or husbands or close friends. In the most optimistic calculations, the costs to save one year of life in patients with CHD has been estimated to be about $10,000, and much more for healthy individuals.

This may not sound unreasonable. Isn't a human life worth $10,000 or more?

The implication of such reasoning is that to add as many years as possible, more than half of mankind should take statin drugs every day from an early age to the end of life. It is easy to calculate that the costs for such treatment would consume most of any government's health budget. And if money is spent to give statin treatment to all healthy people, what will remain for the care of those who really need it? Shouldn't health care be given primarily to the sick and the crippled?

But what is even worse, those who recommend statin treatment for healthy people ignore the fact that the treatment may produce disease instead of preventing it.

Statins produce cancer in animals

Recently, Drs. Thomas Newman and Stephen Hulley from San Francisco published the results of a meticulous review of what we currently know about cancer and cholesterol-lowering drugs. They found that clofibrate (Atromid-S®, Abitrate®), gemfibrozil (Lopid®) and all the statins stimulate cancer growth in rodents.[75]

They asked themselves why these drugs had been approved by the Food and Drug Administration at all. The answer was that the doses used in the animal experiments were much higher than those recommended for clinical use. But as Drs. Newman and Hulley commented, it is more relevant to compare blood levels of the drug. Their review showed that the blood levels that caused cancer in rodents were close to those seen in patients taking the statin drugs.

Because the latent period between exposure to a carcinogen and the incidence of clinical cancer in humans may be 20 years or more, the absence of any controlled trials of this duration means that we do not know whether statin treatment will lead to an increased rate of cancer in coming decades. Thus, millions of healthy people are being treated with medications the ultimate effects of which are not yet known. Drs. Newman and Hulley therefore recommended that the new statins should be used only for patients at very high risk for coronary disease, and avoided for individuals with life expectancies of more than ten to twenty years. Healthy people with high cholesterol as their only risk factor belong to the latter category. Yet these are the very people targeted for cholesterol-lowering drugs in the current trend toward mass medication.

There is good reason to exercise caution in the use of the statin drugs because in the CARE study breast cancer was indeed more common among those who took the drug than in the control group. In the treatment group twelve women got breast cancer during the trial, whereas there was only one case in the control group, a difference that is highly statistically significant.

The authors of the CARE report were eager to explain away the increased frequency of breast cancer. "These findings could be an anomaly," they wrote. It is possible that they are right because the expected number of breast cancer cases in the control group, calculated from the frequency normally seen in the population, should have been five cases. Nevertheless, twelve is more than twice as many as five.

In the package insert for statin drugs, you can read about the risk of various less dangerous side effects, although none of these was reported significantly more often in the treatment group. But nothing is mentioned about the possible risk of breast cancer, the only significant side effect.

Effect and side effect

As you can see from Table 6D, the gain in the numbers of fatal heart attacks was 1.1 percent whereas the loss in numbers of breast cancers was 4.2 percent. Calculated in the way trial directors usually do, as relative rather than absolute risk, the difference was even more striking, with 12 percent fewer heart attacks but 1500 percent more breast cancers. However, you will never see side effects calculated in this way—only positive effects. (Unfortunately, the authors did not give the number of fatal heart attacks for each sex. The figures in the table relate to both sexes.)

As you can see, the number of side effects has tremendous importance when it comes to assessing preventive treatments, because the number of patients experiencing side effects easily exceeds the number of prevented heart attacks. Unfortunately this fact is often ignored or—worse—hidden by using the concept of relative risk to make positive effects seem larger than they are while citing side effects in absolute numbers.

Table 6D. Fatal heart attack and breast cancer rates in the CARE trial.[68]

	Number of patients in the pravastatin group	Number of patients in the control group	Relative Risk	Absolute Risk
Death from a heart attack	96 of 2081 (4.6%)	119 of 2078 (5.7%)	-12%	-1.1%
Cases of breast cancer	13 of 290 (4.5%)	1 of 286 (0.3%)	+1500%	+4.2%

Data from the CARE trial.[63]

Another note of caution

To test a drug on many thousands of patients is extremely costly and laborious. The only groups willing to spend several hundred million dollars for such a trial are, of course, the drug companies because the potential for profits is enormous. Naturally, all of the statin trials were sponsored by the company whose drug was tested in the trial. Not only did the companies pay for the necessary meetings, workshops, conferences, speakers' fees and travel expenses for the many hundreds of participating doctors and researchers in each trial, they also offered assistance in the preparation of the trial, the selection of patients and control individuals, the construction and production of the protocols, the monitoring of the results, the cholesterol analyses and the complicated statistical calculations. Can we be totally confident that their vested interests had no influence at all on the outcome of these trials? Can the wolf serve as shepherd?

And were the results really blinded as we have been told? In most of the trials the lipid analyses were said to have been performed at the drug company laboratories, and these results were not released to the doctors and patients throughout the whole trial. But what about the lipid analyses that may have been performed at individual clinics—were they blinded also? When the first favorable results from the trial were announced in the press, for example, how do you think that the participants in the other trials reacted? Wouldn't they have wanted to know whether they were taking the new wonder drug or whether they were taking an ineffective placebo? One easy way to find out was to take a cholesterol test. Almost certainly, all of them knew their cholesterol level at the beginning of the trial. A new cholesterol test would have easily told them to which group they belonged, and even if their trial doctor hadn't analyzed their cholesterol, it would have been easy to have it done somewhere else.

So it is not unreasonable to assume that a substantial proportion of the patients and their doctors knew to which group the participant belonged and such information may have unintentionally influenced the results.

But let us assume that the doctors and the patients were not influenced at all. What about the trial directors? By now you are familiar with the tendency of the previous directors to exaggerate the trivial effects of their treatment and minimize the side effects. In fact, many of these reports do not appear to have been written by scientists in search of the truth and nothing but the truth.

Consider also that positive results are much more rewarding for researchers than negative ones. Researchers who come up with positive results, in particular, positive results from drug trials, are more often invited as speakers to meetings and congresses and more often chosen for further lucrative research projects.

Should we, therefore, be confident that statin research results have been presented in a nonpartisan manner? Why, for instance, haven't we heard about the outcome of the first statin trial, the EXCEL study?

EXCEL,
the Expanded Clinical Evaluation of Lovastatin

This trial was performed by Dr. Reagan H. Bradford and his group from a large number of American clinics and research institutions, including the Merck Sharp & Dohme Research Laboratories at West Point, NY, where the drug was produced. More than 8000 individuals (called "patients" in the trial reports) with cholesterol levels between 240 and 300 mg/dl received one of four different doses of lovastatin (Mevacor®) or a placebo.

With a view to reporting on possible adverse effects of the treatment, preliminary study results were published after only one year of the trial.[76] No significant side effects were reported, but in the fine print the authors were obliged to mention that death due to all causes was 0.5 percent in the four lovastatin groups combined (32 or 33 individuals out of a group of about 6600—no exact figures were given in the report) compared to

0.2 percent in the placebo group (three or four individuals out of a group of 1650). By taking all the lovastatin groups together, the difference would have been statistically significant if the number of deaths in the treatment groups were 33, but not if it were 32. Even if the difference were not statistically significant after one year, it would certainly have become significant if the tendency to a higher mortality in the treatment groups had continued throughout the trial. In any case, the aim of the treatment was to lower mortality and most certainly no lowering was achieved.

Today at least 20 reports from the EXCEL trial have been published in various medical journals. These reports tell us how well lovastatin is tolerated and how effective it is in lowering blood cholesterol levels in various populations, but not one of them has reported the final outcome of the trial, although more than ten years have passed since it began. Therefore, we do not know whether the increased mortality, seen after just one year of treatment, has continued throughout the trial.

Why, then, have we never heard about the outcome of the first statin trial, which was one of the largest?[77] And are there more trials we haven't heard about? Or are there any unfavorable effects in the published trials that we haven't heard about either?

It is safe to assume that it is not a harmless enterprise to lower cholesterol by drugs. And other unpleasant things may happen to you if you follow the advice of the diet-heart proponents. More about that in the next chapter.

New guidelines

On May 16, 2001 an expert panel from the National Cholesterol Education Program published new guidelines for "the detection, evaluation and treatment of high blood cholesterol."[78] The guidelines are designed to convert healthy people into patients and put most of mankind on cholesterol-lowering diets and drugs.

The guidelines introduce new risk factors that demand preventive measures (or "risk-reduction therapy," as they call it) and widen the limits for the old ones.

The main target is LDL-cholesterol, because "research from experimental animals, laboratory investigations, epidemiology, and genetic forms of hypercholesterolemia indicate that elevated LDL-cholesterol is a major cause of CHD." (If you have read this book from the beginning you will probably agree with me that such research has indicated nothing of the kind.) The optimal values are 150 for LDL and 200 for total cholesterol. But if there are any risk factors present, the optimal cholesterol level should be lowered, say the guidelines. The more risk factors, the lower cholesterol should be.

In the highest risk category are patients with coronary heart disease because, according to the statistics from Framingham, they run more than a 20 percent risk of having a new heart attack in ten years. (We are not told where to find these figures, however.) Other atherosclerotic disease is said to be just as risky, such as is diabetes from the age of twenty. The presence of two or more other serious risk factors is said to put the patient at a similar risk.

The new guidelines provide an intricate scoring system showing how the different risk factors are graded. Men with an accumulated score of 15 or more belong to the highest risk category. And it is easy to get a high score. For instance, if you are seventy years old, you are automatically given 12 points. A cholesterol level above 275 at age 39 gives you 11 points, less with increasing age. An untreated systolic blood pressure reading of 130 (which is completely normal) gets one point; if you are being treated for high blood pressure and your reading is 130, you get two points.

Smokers below age 40 get eight points—and you are a smoker if you have smoked at least one cigarette during the last month. Women need a higher score to be placed in the highest risk category—but they get more points for their risk factors.

The guidelines recommend that everybody over age 20 have his or her cholesterol levels tested every fifth year. If you are in the highest risk category and your LDL-cholesterol is above 100, you should change your life habits; if your LDL is above 130, you should immediately take a cholesterol-lowering drug. But you might as well start with both measures, say the guidelines, because few people succeed in lowering their cholesterol by life-habit intervention alone. (Elsewhere in the paper the authors claim that life-habit intervention is an effective way of lowering cholesterol!)

Emerging risk factors

The indications for treatment are stronger if there are other risk factors than those mentioned above, for instance if you are overweight, if you don't exercise or if you eat too much animal fat. Even "emerging" risk factors should be taken into consideration, and by emerging risk factors the authors include almost all laboratory tests that, on average, have been found higher in patients with heart disease. According to the authors, "the emerging risk factors do not categorically modify LDL-cholesterol goals; however, they appear to contribute to CHD risk to varying degrees and can have utility in selected persons to guide intensity of risk-reduction therapy." (In other words, take a bunch of laboratory tests and most of us become candidates for statin treatment.)

Subclinical atherosclerosis

One of the emerging risk factors is called "subclinical atherosclerotic disease." The guidelines give no explanation for this new concept. The term comes from a new technique called electron beam tomography which is a method for depicting calcifications in the coronary arteries from the outside. The degree of calcification is said to reflect the degree of atherosclerosis and is therefore a much better predictor of future heart attack than high blood cholesterol or, for that matter, any other risk factor. According to an advertisement for one of those huge health centers that have become popular in the US, "The electron beam tomography scan gives individuals who have risk factors for heart disease a painless, non-invasive way to obtain peace of mind knowing that early indications of heart disease are or are not present."

Whether you obtain any peace of mind is questionable because in the most recent study using electron beam tomography, sixty percent of a group of healthy women over age 55 had "subclinical atherosclerosis;" yet, according to the new guidelines, half of these women belonged to the low-risk category.[79] In other words, with one blow this new technique has landed many further millions of people into the high-risk category.

The most surprising finding, at least for those who have not read Chapter 4, was the lack of an association between degree of calcification and total or LDL-cholesterol or any other lipid fraction. The authors of the study had no comments about this finding—which is totally devastating to the cholesterol hypothesis—except to say that they considered the new guidelines insufficient and suggested regular electron beam tomography for the whole population.

More new risk factors

The guidelines state officially for the first time that high triglycerides should be lowered and low HDL-cholesterol should be raised. True enough, admit the authors, it has never been proved that raising HDL-cholesterol provides any benefit. (There is no evidence that lowering triglycerides provides any benefit either.) Nevertheless, they recommend treatment with clofibrate (Atromid-S®, Abitrate®) or nicotinic acid (niacin). Obviously, the many unsuccessful trials with these drugs, and their many harmful side effects, are completely forgotten.

The dietary recommendations—changed for at least the seventh time since the 1960s—include a substantial increase in carbohydrate consumption. The bedeviling inconsistencies of the dietary recommendations thus appear in full daylight, as a diet rich in carbohydrates is well known to lower HDL-cholesterol and to raise triglycerides. Not that such changes matter in themselves, but as the panel considers "abnormal" values of these lipids to be dangerous, the advice is of course contradictory.

Evidently, the advice is directed to diabetic patients also, because no specific dietary recommendations are given for that category of human beings. But to suggest that diabetic patients should obtain a large percentage of their caloric intake from carbohydrates seems unusually bad advice. Most carbohydrates are quickly transformed into glucose inducing rapid changes in blood glucose and insulin levels and thus stimulating a conversion of blood glucose to depot fat and chronic feelings of hunger.

A new risk factor, considered just as dangerous as heart disease, is called the "metabolic syndrome." According to the authors, you are suffering from the metabolic syndrome if you have three or more of the risk factors mentioned below:

Table 6E. The New Guidelines

Risk factor	Definition according to the new guidelines
Abdominal obesity	Waist circumference: men: >40 inches* women: >35 inches
High blood pressure	>135/85 mm
High triglycerides	>150mg/dl
Low HDL-cholesterol	men: <40 mg/dl women: <50 mg/dl
High fasting blood sugar	110-125 mg/dl

*A waist circumference above 40 inches is considered harmful for some male "patients." Nothing is said about what is meant by "some."

Test yourself and your family! You'll find that most of you "suffer" from the metabolic syndrome. And this combination or risk factors, says the panel, conveys the same high risk for future heart disease as having already had a heart attack!

It has been calculated that, were the new guidelines followed consistently, the number of people in need of cholesterol-lowering drugs would increase from 13 to 36 million people, or 18 percent of the adult population. Even this high figure is a serious underestimation. If the new guidelines are correct, then the majority of the human race needs life-habit intervention. But to change one's life habits is notoriously difficult and as such measures are rarely followed by any substantial cholesterol lowering either, the list of candidates for drug treatment seems almost endless.

But isn't it true that a stitch in time saves nine? Aren't these guidelines a glorious yet harmless way to prevent cardiovascular death in a large number of human beings? Isn't it true, as stated to the press by Claude Lenfant, Director of the National Heart, Lung and Blood Institute, that "the statins dramatically reduce a person's risk for CHD"?

If you have read this book from the beginning you already know the answer, but let's review the "dramatic" effect of statin treatment.

As an argument for using cholesterol-lowering drugs, the authors claim that 20 percent of patients with coronary heart disease have a new heart attack after ten years. But that number is obtained by including minor symptoms without any clinical significance. Most people survive even a major heart attack, many with few or no symptoms after recovery. Heart attacks may even appear without any symptoms. I have seen many patients myself with indisputable electrocardiographic indications of a recent myocardial infarction, but without recalling more than slight discomfort, if any symptoms at all, during the preceding weeks. What matters is how many die and this is much less than 20 percent. For instance, look at Table 6C on page 202. Here you will see that in the trials that included patients with heart disease, the risk of dying from a heart attack in 5-6 years was between 5.7 and 8.5 percent. And for healthy people with high cholesterol, it was less than 1 percent. Or, put in another way, the chance for a healthy individual with high cholesterol of not dying from a heart attack in 5-6 years was 98.4 percent, a chance you could improve to 98.8 percent with statin treatment.

In conclusion, the new guidelines may possibly prevent cardiovascular death in a small minority of patients with cardiovascular disease. But at the same time they may increase mortality from other diseases, transform healthy individuals into unhappy hypochondriacs obsessed with the chemical composition of their food and their blood, reduce the income of ranchers and dairy farmers, undermine the art of cuisine, destroy the joy of eating, and divert health care money from the sick and the poor to the rich and the healthy. The only winners are the drug companies and imitation food industry, and the researchers that they support.[80]

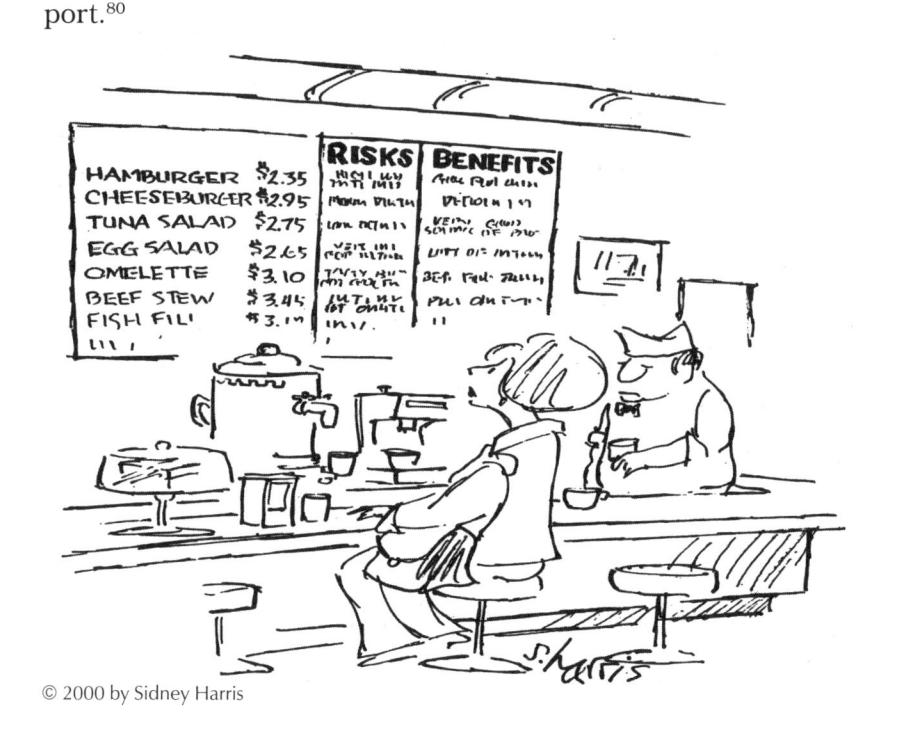

DR. ORNISH AND
THE LIFESTYLE HEART TRIAL

Coronary heart disease is a multifactorial disease that requires multifactorial intervention. This is the view of Dr. Dean Ornish and his group at the Preventive Medicine Research Institute, Sausalito, California, a view they share with many other doctors and researchers. Dr. Ornish and his group chose to intervene with a low-fat, low-cholesterol vegetarian diet, smoking cessation, stress-management training and moderate exercise. They selected 94 patients with a diagnosis of coronary artery disease according to a previous coronary angiogram. Fifty-three were randomly assigned to the experimental group and 43 to the control group, but when told about the design of the study only 28 and 20, respectively, agreed to participate.

A new angiogram was performed after one year, but one of the angiograms disappeared; in three patients the second angiogram could not be evaluated; one patient was not studied because of unpaid bills; one died during heavy exercise; and one dropped out because of alcohol misuse. Thus, only 22 patients in the experimental group and nineteen in the control group were available for analysis.

The result seemed promising. In the treatment group the total cholesterol fell by an average of 24 percent and LDL-cholesterol by 37 percent; mean body weight had decreased by ten kilograms; less severe chest pains were reported; and the coronary arteries had widened a little, whereas they had become a little more narrow in the control group. These improvements were strongly related to the degree of adherence to the intervention program in a "dose-response" manner, as the authors wrote in their report. The vascular improvements were still there after a prolongation of the study by five years, but now the difference was calculated using the less-demanding one-tailed t-test. Unfor-

tunately, there was no difference in frequency, duration or severity of angina between the groups, but this unexpected finding was
"most likely" due to bypass operations performed in the control
group. Nothing was mentioned about how many operations had
been performed, however, and no comparison was made between those who had not had an operation. In addition, a further
six individuals were unavailable for follow-up study.

And there were more flaws. Not only was it an unblinded study
(although in the latest publication it was called blinded!), the low
number of participants also resulted in a most uneven distribution
of the risk factors. For instance, at the start the mean age was four
years higher, mean total cholesterol 8 percent higher and mean
LDL-cholesterol 10 percent higher in the control group; but mean
body weight was almost 25 pounds higher in the treatment group.
Such large differences between risk factors obviously complicate
the evaluation of the treatment effect.

But let us assume that the improvement of the treated individuals was true and a result of the intervention—and this may well be
possible—which of the intervention measures had a beneficial effect? Was it a weight reduction of more than 25 pounds? Was it a
difference in smoking habits? (One in the experimental group
smoked and stopped; nothing was mentioned about the number
of smokers in the control group.) Was it the exercise? Was it the
inner sense of peace and well-being produced by the stress-management education? Or was it a combination of these factors?

That the diet had any importance is unlikely because there is
little evidence that vegetarians have a lower risk of coronary disease than other people.[81] (See page 109.) It is also unlikely that it
was the change of LDL-cholesterol because at the end of the study
there were no significant differences between these values in the
two groups. The latter also contradicts the statement that the changes
of coronary atherosclerosis and the diet were strongly correlated in a
"dose-response" manner. To the pertinent question "Precisely

how strong were the correlations?" asked by Elaine R. Monsen, editor of *Journal of the American Dietetic Association*, Dr. Ornish answered that "the study wasn't really set up to do these kinds of analyses, so when we get beyond saying they're correlated, we're on shaky ground."

It is laudable to try prevention without drugs, and we already know that it may be health-promoting to avoid being overweight, to exercise a little and to avoid smoking and mental stress, but with such weak evidence, why inflict a diet that only rabbits may find tolerable on millions of people? Perhaps the results would have been better if the patients' inner sense of peace and well-being had been strengthened even further by allowing them to eat more satisfying and nutritious food.

(Ornish D and others. Can lifestyle changes reverse coronary heart disease? The Lifestyle Heart Trial. *The Lancet* 336, 129-133, 1990; Ornish D. Reversing heart disease through diet, exercise and stress management: An interview with Dean Ornish. *Journal of the American Dietetic Association* 91, 162-165, 1991; Gould KL, Ornish D and others. Changes in myocardial perfusion abnormalities by positron emission tomography after long-term, intense risk factor modification. *Journal of the American Medical Association* 274, 894-901, 1995)

Myth 7

Polyunsaturated Oils are Good for You

Intervening is a way of causing trouble.

Lewis Thomas

Risk at both ends of the scale

The smaller number of heart disease deaths in the Veterans Administration soybean trial, mentioned in Chapter 6, was off-set by a larger number of cancer deaths. Does this mean that soybean oil causes cancer?

Diet-heart proponents would argue that Dr. Dayton's soybean trial was an anomaly, and that other trials with polyunsaturated oils have not resulted in more cancer. However, never before have such huge amounts of polyunsaturated oil been consumed over such a long period of time. Dr. Dayton's patients were also much older than in the other trials, and thus more susceptible to cancer, which means that a possible cancer-provoking effect could be detected more easily.

Another disquieting fact is that many studies have reported low cholesterol to be a risk factor for cancer. The purpose of these studies was to follow a great number of individuals for many years to see whether the Framingham researchers were right when they claimed that high cholesterol means a high risk of heart attack. Surprisingly, these more recent studies revealed that it was just as dangerous to have a very low cholesterol level as it was to have a very high one. Those who had very low levels of cholesterol had a greater incidence of cancer while those with very high cholesterol suffered more heart attacks.[1]

Most investigators thought that low cholesterol levels were not the cause but the *result* of cancer since cancer cells need cholesterol, just as any other cells do. Perhaps their rapid growth and greater need for cholesterol reduced the cholesterol levels in the blood?

It is interesting that the diet-heart proponents immediately relegate low blood cholesterol to a secondary and thus an innocent phenomenon in the etiology of cancer, but never admit that high cholesterol might be a secondary and thus innocent phenomenon in the etiology of heart disease. No, say the diet-heart proponents, high cholesterol is always dangerous and should be lowered by any means.

A great number of studies also found that cholesterol tends

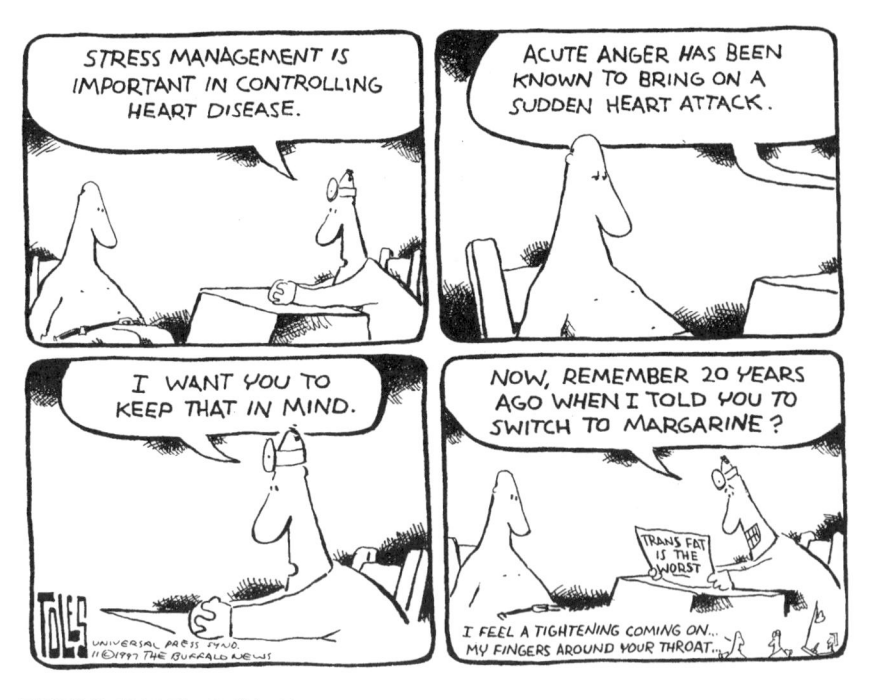

TOLES © 1997 The Buffalo News.

to be low many years before cancer is discovered.[1] If low cholesterol was a consequence of rapid cancer growth, then the level should decrease when the cancer started to grow substantially. But in some patients cholesterol was low 18 years before the cancer appeared.

Of course, this fact was a serious drawback for those who planned cholesterol-lowering measures for most of the population, and the diet-heart proponents therefore met in 1981 to discuss the problem.[2]

The meeting was of sufficient importance to attract most of the leading American cholesterol researchers, including Chicago professor Jeremiah Stamler, director of two major cholesterol-lowering trials and author of a large number of papers that expanded on the dangers of high cholesterol; Basil Rifkind, head of the Lipid Metabolism Branch at the National Heart, Lung and Blood Institute and later head of the LRC trial; Robert Levy from Columbia University, chairman of the meeting and previously director of the National Heart, Lung and Blood Institute; Antonio Gotto, director of the American Heart Association; Ancel Keys; and many more of those who made up the anti-cholesterol army.

Predictably, the participants concluded that low cholesterol did not cause cancer, but they were unable to explain the phenomenon. It was a subject for further research, they noted, but not a threat to public health.

The published report from the meeting stated: "It was a unanimous opinion of the panelists that the data did not preclude, countermand, or contradict the current public health message which recommends that those with elevated cholesterol levels seek to lower them. There is evidence of a possible increase in cancer risk at very low cholesterol levels (but) the risk is generally modest."[3]

These were their words. By "very low levels" the panel meant less than 183 mg/dl. But diet-heart proponents do not consider 183 mg/dl too low when it comes to treatment of high cholesterol. A couple of years later, for instance, members of the National Heart, Lung and Blood Institute and the American Heart Association (many of whom participated in the meeting) recommended that people should bring their cholesterol levels down to at least 190 mg/dl.

It is not certain that low cholesterol levels provoke cancer: the fact that cancer is seen more often in individuals with low cholesterol is not proof of cause and effect. Low cholesterol is a risk factor for cancer, precisely as high cholesterol is a risk factor for heart disease. Again, a risk factor is not necessarily the cause. Something may produce cancer and at the same time lower blood cholesterol. Chemical compounds with such a potential do exist.

Burglars among molecules

"Somewhere, on some remote planet. . . on the other side of our galaxy, there is at this moment a committee nearing the end of a year-long study of our own tiny, provincial solar system. The intelligent beings of that place are putting their signatures. . . to a paper which asserts, with finality, that life is out of the question here and the place is not worth an expedition. Their instruments have detected the presence of that most lethal of all gases, oxygen, and that is the end of that."

With these words Lewis Thomas, famous essayist and professor of medicine, opened one of his lectures to his new students. Thomas used his story to illustrate another point. But his fantasy was not created out of thin air—oxygen is dangerous.

A civil war rages inside us from the sweet second of fecundation until we end as dust or ashes. Atoms and molecules are fighting for the tiny elements that are surrounding them, the electrons. The haze of electrons gives identity and character to each atom and molecule; if the number of electrons is altered, a valuable molecular citizen may, in a split second, be turned into a useless and even destructive hoodlum.

Electrons prefer to be present as couples. Paired electrons furnish the atom or molecule with stability and resistance against harassment, but some pairs are more stable than others.

The main part of a fatty acid is composed of a core of carbon atoms to which hydrogen atoms are attached. When the number of hydrogen atoms is optimal, their electrons form stable pairs with those of the carbon atoms. Examples of stable molecules are the saturated fatty acids, those said to be dangerous to the heart and the vessels. They are called saturated because they are saturated with hydrogen.

Unsaturated fatty acids are missing hydrogen atoms. Monounsaturated fatty acids are missing two atoms, polyunsaturated fatty acids are missing four or more. This means that instead of sharing one pair of electrons with each other, some of the carbon atoms are sharing two pairs of electrons with their neighbor carbon instead of one pair, forming the so-called double bond. A double bond is less stable than a single bond. A hydrogen atom sitting close to a double bond is easily snatched by a free radical. Free radicals snatch hydrogen atoms because one or more of their electrons lack their partner; they are unpaired.

Combustion fumes, such as cigarette smoke and diesel exhaust, are especially rich in free radicals, but even the oxygen molecule is a free radical.[4] It is especially active when heated. If the temperature is high enough, all its susceptible neighbors are oxidized—they burn. But what we are interested in here is oxidation at body temperature.

Inside the cells of our body oxidation is vital to cell function and life as long as this process is controlled by hormones and enzymes. Step by step, sugar and other fuel molecules are oxidized to water and carbon dioxide, a process that releases energy for the cell machinery. So far so good.

But if oxidation occurs without control, as it may do if we are exposed to free radicals, molecules other than sugar may be oxidized. Among these others are the unstable polyunsaturated fatty acids. Loss of hydrogen atoms is disastrous to a polyunsaturated fatty acid (as to other molecules as well), because its stability is ruined and it is oxidized or split into lesser molecules with nasty qualities.

Usually the human body is protected against oxidation thanks to many various antioxidants, kind molecules that donate hydrogen atoms to the free radicals, thus protecting us against uncontrolled oxidation. Vitamin E, for example, is a well-known and important antioxidant that protects the polyunsaturated fatty aids in our cell membranes. There are many others.

But if too many polyunsaturated fatty acids are present, or if too many free radicals are available, or if the amount of antioxidants is insufficient, then the antioxidants may fail to protect the body.

Nobody knows the limit between harmless and harmful amounts of polyunsaturated fatty acids in the diet. Cholesterol campaigners now recommend no more than 10 per cent of our calories from polyunsaturated oils, but give no reasons for the limit. They don't tell us about the evidence that an excess of dietary polyunsaturated fatty acids may be dangerous.[5]

Does polyunsaturated oil produce cancer?

When too much polyunsaturated oil is given to laboratory animals, their white blood cells become damaged so that the animals die more easily from infectious diseases and cancer. We do not know for sure whether the same is valid for human beings, but we do know that our immune system is sensitive to a surplus of polyunsaturated fatty acids. If a preparation of such oils is added to the diet of patients who have received a kidney graft, the function of their white blood cells is hampered, resulting in a better acceptance of foreign material, including the transplanted kidney.[6]

But other foreign and less useful material, such as bacteria and viruses, may also be accepted. One of the great problems with transplant patients is that their immunosuppressive treatment makes them more vulnerable to infection. It is a general rule that any substance that harms the white blood cells also stimulates infection. Some of these substances may even stimulate cancer.

It has not yet been definitely proven that polyunsaturated fatty acids stimulate cancer in human beings, but proof may come in time. By analogy, cigarette smoke may produce cancer, but only after many years of smoking.

Today most deep-frying is done in vegetable oils. Very few know that if polyunsaturated fatty acids are kept hot over many hours, their tendency to produce cancer in laboratory animals increases.[7]

Do polyunsaturated oils make you age faster?

It is commonly accepted that aging is partly a result of the eternal fight of free radicals for hydrogen atoms. If laboratory animals are exposed to free radicals, or to substances highly sensitive to free radicals—if, for instance, these animals eat large amounts of polyunsaturated oils—yellowish pigments are stored in many organs. The same pigments develop in most creatures, including man, and accumulate with age.

The fact that polyunsaturated oils may accelerate aging was demonstrated by Dr. Edward Pinckney. (See Chapter 9.) In collaboration with a plastic surgeon, he asked a large number of patients how much polyunsaturated oil they usually consumed.

Fifty-four percent of the patients said that they had increased their intake considerably. Of those patients, 78 percent showed marked clinical signs of premature aging, and 60 percent had required the removal of one or more skin lesions because of suspected malignancy. Of the patients who had made no special efforts to consume polyunsaturated oils, the figures were 18 and 8 percent respectively.[5b]

Do polyunsaturated oils make you stupid?

Polyunsaturates have other nasty effects. Premature children have only small amounts of vitamin E in their bodies. Dr. Joshua Ritchie and his team in San Francisco studied seven premature babies who were admitted to the hospital with widespread edema, anemia, disturbances of the blood cells and lack of vitamin E. The researchers found that the most plausible cause was the food; these children had all received commercial formulas composed of skim milk and vegetable oils with a high content of polyunsaturated fatty acids.[8]

The brain has low levels of vitamin E. This fact may explain why chickens fed polyunsaturated oil develop brain damage very quickly.[9]

Do polyunsaturated oils cause atherosclerosis?

A new theory about the origin of atherosclerosis is that it is not normal cholesterol, but oxidized cholesterol that is dangerous.[10] And oxidized cholesterol means cholesterol that has been damaged by free radicals.

Even in the fetus the artery walls are speckled with fat. The microscope shows that these speckles or fatty streaks are composed of white blood cells filled with tiny bubbles. These cells are called foam cells. But the substance is not foam; it is cholesterol.

Patients with homozygous familial hypercholesterolemia have foam cells also. This fact was a stumbling block to the Nobel Prize winners Michael Brown and Joseph Goldstein. What they discovered was that in individuals with the rare genetic error called familial hypercholesterolemia, cholesterol molecules in the blood do not enter the cells as they do in normal individuals. The reason is that the key to the cell, the so-called LDL-receptor, is defective. Individuals who have inherited the disease from one parent (heterozygous form) have too few receptors; those who have inherited the disease from both parents (homozygous form) have no receptors at all. The lack of LDL-receptors explains why patients with familial hypercholesterolemia have such high levels of cholesterol in their blood—anywhere from 350 mg/dl all the way up to 1000 mg/dl.

But how can cholesterol enter the foam cells in patients with the homozygous form of familial hypercholesterolemia if, as Brown and Goldstein suggested, the cholesterol door to the cell is closed? This is certainly a crucial question because diet-heart proponents consider these foam cells the forerunner of atherosclerosis.

Recent studies have shown that it is not normal cholesterol that accumulates in the foam cells but oxidized cholesterol. And oxidized cholesterol has no problem entering the cells; it takes another route. The problem seemed solved.

But how does cholesterol become oxidized?

There is a large body of evidence indicating that free radicals are the cause of the oxidation, and the source of free radicals is most probably the polyunsaturated vegetable oils. For example, scientists can reduce the fatty streaks (called athero-sclerosis by the proponents) in rabbits with familial hyper-cholesterolemia[11] (named Watanabe rabbits) with the drug probucol, which in rabbits does not lower blood cholesterol.[12] The explanation may be that probucol, just like vitamin E, is an antioxidant that hampers the attacks of free radicals.

On the other hand, lowering cholesterol in Watanabe rabbits does not reduce the fatty streaks.[13]

If polyunsaturated fatty acids promote oxidation of cholesterol and thus atherosclerosis, we should avoid eating too much of them. But diet-heart proponents continue to insist that it is more important to lower cholesterol by avoiding saturated fat, and continue to recommend polyunsaturates as a substitute.

It is difficult to follow the proponents' line of thought. The deposition of cholesterol in the artery walls of Watanabe rabbits was not reduced by lowering the blood cholesterol but by preventing its oxidation. Why, then, do they recommend more polyunsaturated oils if too much of it stimulates oxidation?

Dr. Daniel Steinberg from the University of California at La Jolla has played an important role in introducing the new theory about oxidized cholesterol. He was chairman of the consensus committee that started the National Cholesterol Education Program. This campaign has recommended that all Americans consume polyunsaturated vegetable oils instead of saturated fat.

The committee recommended an upper limit of 10 percent for the consumption of polyunsaturated oil (and now the reader knows why). However, the committee did not call attention to the fact that the food they had previously called a protection against atherosclerosis was now seen as its cause.

It has not been definitely proven, however, that oxidized cholesterol is the forerunner of atherosclerosis. A link is missing.

What has been demonstrated is that oxidized cholesterol is accumulated as fatty streaks, but the presence of fatty streaks is not the same as atherosclerosis. And the accumulation of cholesterol in fatty streaks has been shown in Watanabe rabbits, not in common rabbits. Because Watanabe rabbits inherit the same defect in cholesterol metabolism as people with familial hypercholesterolemia, the correct conclusion from the rabbit experiments may be that fatty streaks in individuals with familial hypercholesterolemia are induced by oxidized cholesterol.

However, there are observations that do suggest an adverse effect of polyunsaturated oils on atherosclerosis. In the world-wide epidemiological study of atherosclerosis (see Chapter 1), the investigators found a connection between the degree of atherosclerosis and the total intake of fat. As there was no association between the intake of saturated fat and degree of atherosclerosis, the association obviously concerned unsaturated fats. (However, as mentioned before, a mere association does not prove that unsaturated fat promotes atherosclerosis, but the observation definitely contradicts the notion that saturated fat does.)

What we know for certain is that polyunsaturated fatty acids may produce a great many unfortunate effects, none of them pleasant for human beings. We need polyunsaturated fats in small amounts to keep us healthy; some of them are even essential to life. Thanks to their lack of hydrogen atoms, polyunsaturated fatty acids are soft and flexible. If our cell walls contained only saturated fats, we would probably become as stiff as candles. An excess of dietary polyunsaturated fatty acids, however, is undesirable. After all, who wants his home to be occupied by terrorists?[14]

Trans fat

The fact that polyunsaturated fats such as corn, soybean and sunflower oils are liquid, even at cold temperatures, has been a problem for the oil manufacturers in countries where butter and lard, and not vegetable oils, were traditionally used in the diet. Vegetable oils cannot be spread on bread, give unsatisfactory results in baking and produce burnt and rancid smells when used for frying.

However, early in this century French and German food technologists invented a method for converting liquid vegetable oil into solid fat. They heated the oil to 300-400° Fahrenheit in large reactors, mixed the oil with nickel powder that acted as a catalyst and then forced hydrogen through this unappetizing soup. This method, still used today, changes the chemical structure of the polyunsaturated fatty acids and creates something called *trans* fatty acids. *Trans* fatty acids are also unsaturated, but the hydrogen molecules in the double bonds have been rearranged so that the resulting molecules behave like the more solid saturated fatty acids. The final product, which is a mixture of various polyunsaturated, saturated and *trans* fatty acids, is called partially hydrogenated oil and is used as an ingredient in many food products including margarine, crackers, cookies, doughnuts, french fries, potato chips, pastries and sweets.

Tiny amounts of a certain type of *trans* fatty acid are also found in animal fats. However, the kinds of *trans* fatty acids that are produced by industrial hydrogenation are rarely found in natural food. Unfortunately, the body doesn't recognize the unnatural *trans* fatty acids found in modern foods as foreign. Instead of rejecting them, the body builds these manufactured fats with their misplaced electrons into the cell walls and other parts of human cells, leading to disturbances in cellular function if we eat too much of them.[15]

There are polyunsaturated fatty acids that we cannot synthesize ourselves but must obtain in small amounts from our food. These essential fatty acids (EFAs), as they are called, are vital, just as vitamins are. Normally, the risk of suffering from lack of essential fatty acids is small because they are found naturally in most foods. However, when experimental animals are fed *trans* fatty acids from the partial hydrogenation process, they develop symptoms similar to those of essential fatty acid deficiency, either because the *trans* fatty acids are toxic by themselves or because, in some way, they inhibit use of the essential fatty acids. The most serious effects concern reproduction. The testicles of rats are damaged, and the rats become sterile;[16] in mice, the fat content of the milk decreases.[17] In human beings, *trans* fatty acids in the mother's blood pass over to the fetus. The research of Dr. B. Koletzko at the Pediatric Department at Ludwig-Maximilians University in Munich, who studied premature infants, suggests that *trans* fats in the mother's diet may have an effect on the health of the fetus. He found that low birth weight in these children was associated with a higher proportion of *trans* fatty acids in the blood.[18]

Of course, this is no proof that the low birth weight of these children was due to the excess of *trans* fatty acids, but the finding certainly gives rise for concern because there is experimental evidence that *trans* fatty acids may inhibit growth. This was discovered in a study by Dr. S. Atal and his co-workers at various institutions at the University of Maryland and at the National Institutes of Health.[19] They gave young mice two different diets. The only difference between the diets was that a tiny amount of normal fatty acids (not of the essential ones) was substituted with the same amount of *trans* fatty acids. After two years the body weight of the mice fed with *trans* fatty acids was 20-25 percent lower than the weight of the control mice. Thus, although the mice had received exactly the same amount of calories, those who got *trans* fatty acids instead of other naturally occurring fatty acids did not grow as they should have.

Too much dietary *trans* fat makes the blood cholesterol level rise.[20] Not that this effect matters much in itself; if you haven't skipped Chapter 4, you may recall that atherosclerosis has nothing to do with the blood cholesterol level, and from Chapter 2 you may remember that most heart attacks are seen in people with normal cholesterol levels. But people who think that the cholesterol level is important should know that by following the official recommendations and eating margarine rather than animal fats, they may raise their cholesterol instead of lowering it.

Trans fat is present in considerable amounts in solid margarine and in bakery shortenings. The consumption of *trans* fat has increased substantially in most Western countries during the last century. In the United States, a rough estimate is an increase from about 12 grams per day per person before World War II to about 40 grams in 1985.[15] This is the average figure; some people consume far greater quantities, especially if they have followed the recommendations of the National Cholesterol Education Program, because very often fat that is called polyunsaturated on the food labels may actually be *trans* fat, and foods labeled "low-fat" may in fact contain large amounts of fat, particularly *trans* fat. Even the few people who prefer butter over margarine consume *trans* fat if they eat processed food products such as crackers, cookies, chips, french fries and baked goods.

"First do no harm," said Hippocrates. Many researchers, in particular those who advocate the diet-heart idea, argue that the evidence implicating *trans* fats as harmful is weak. However, the mere suspicion that reproduction and growth may be hampered by an unnatural food component, or that the same component may stimulate cancer growth, demands that it be subjected to thorough scientific scrutiny. Instead *trans* fats have silently infiltrated the food supply, like a marauder in the night.

And there are still more drawbacks associated with lowering blood cholesterol.

"Unlikely effects"

In several of the trials described in Chapter 6, a larger number of the treated individuals died from violence or suicide. In the LRC trial there were eleven such deaths compared to four in the control group; in the first trial from Helsinki, there were four compared to one; in the second trial, there were ten compared to four; in the Oslo trial, three compared to one; in the Upjohn trial, two compared to zero; in the 1978 WHO trial, eighteen compared to fifteen; in the Veterans Administration trial with soybean oil, four compared to zero; in the Minnesota trial, twenty-one compared to fourteen; in Miettinen's trial, four compared to zero. In none of these studies was the difference statistically significant, but all the studies pointed in the same direction.

Most diet-heart proponents belittle this problem. It must be coincidental, they say. It is out of the question, they say, that lowering cholesterol makes people more likely to die from violence or suicide.

Matthew Muldoon, assistant professor in the Department of Medicine; Stephen Manuck, professor in the Department of Psychology; and Karen Matthews, professor in the Department of Psychiatry, University of Pittsburgh, Pennsylvania, were the first to point out this phenomenon.[21] Their conclusion was that if all the results were added up in a meta-analysis, the number who died from violence and suicide was, in fact, statistically significant. These researchers also showed that the rate of death from violence and suicide in the control groups was identical with the rate in the whole US, while the rate was twice as great in the treatment groups. They also calculated that the "profit" in numbers of fatal heart attacks in the treatment groups was 28 lives, while the "loss" from violent and sudden death was 29 lives (both figures per 100,000).

The Pittsburgh investigators were not surprised. One of them had previously given the diet recommended by the cholesterol campaign to apes and had found that the animals became more aggressive than apes fed cholesterol and animal fat.

Professor Muldoon and his associates also stressed that low blood cholesterol levels are more often observed in criminals, people with diagnoses of violent or aggressive-conduct disorders, homicidal offenders with histories of violence and suicide attempts related to alcohol, and people with poorly internalized social norms and low self-control.

In a comment on the paper of Muldoon and associates, David Horrobin, the editor of *Medical Hypotheses*, said that the most serious consequence of lowering blood cholesterol is invisible. If low cholesterol levels cause violence and depression, then intervention to reduce cholesterol on a large scale could lead to a general shift to more violent patterns of behavior. Most of this increased violence would not result in death but in more aggression at work and in the family, more child abuse, more wife-beating and generally more unhappiness. Such events are not recorded in the trials, and they are therefore never detected.[22]

In other words, we are told about the number surviving a heart attack, but not about the number surviving violence or suicide attempts.

The conclusions of Muldoon and co-workers were strengthened by a large investigation in Sweden by Dr. Gunnar Lindberg and colleagues.[23] They measured blood cholesterol levels in more than 50,000 men and women and then kept track of them for 20 years. During the first six years, 20 men with cholesterol below 207 mg/dl (those in the first quartile), but only five with cholesterol above 296 mg/dl (those in the fourth quartile) had committed suicide.

The increased risk of suicide disappeared with time. The authors therefore concluded that the increased risk of suicide may be associated with a concentration of cholesterol below a subject's habitual value, which means that the risk of suicide is greater if the low cholesterol is induced by diet or drugs. They found no increased risk for women, but their number of suicides was much smaller.

Recently, Dr. Beatrice Golomb at the University of California at Los Angeles reported a meticulous analysis of all studies published since 1965 that looked at the association between low or lowered cholesterol levels and violence. She concluded that the association is causal, and that the risk of creating violent behavior should be taken in consideration before doctors advise their patients to lower cholesterol.[24]

Nothing to be afraid of

In Japan, more people die from cerebral hemorrhage (stroke due to bleeding from a cerebral artery) than in most other countries, a fact that is never mentioned when the benefits of the lean Japanese diet, their low cholesterol and their low coronary mortality are emphasized. The risk of dying from a cerebral hemorrhage is greatest for Japanese with low blood cholesterol levels. Diet-heart proponents never mention this fact either, or they say that it is something peculiar to the Japanese.

Cerebral hemorrhage is not a common cause of death among middle-aged men in the West; for every death due to a cerebral hemorrhage, there are ten from coronary heart disease. It is therefore necessary to study a great many individuals to determine any possible connection between the blood cholesterol levels and the risk of cerebral hemorrhage. One such study exists.

Before the start of MRFIT, blood cholesterol was measured in more than 300,000 middle-aged American men, the MRFIT screenees. An investigation six years later showed that the risk of cerebral hemorrhage for people with low blood cholesterol was not peculiar to Japan; the risk was also present in the US, but only in men with elevated blood pressure. Of ten thousand men with high blood pressure, 23 with low blood cholesterol level died from cerebral hemorrhage compared to only four with high cholesterol.[25]

It is interesting to note how anxious the MRFIT investigators were to downplay this fact. The coronary mortality among those with the highest cholesterol values was 242 percent, or 1.3 percentage points greater than for those who had the lowest cholesterol values. But the MRFIT researchers did not calculate the increased risk of cerebral hemorrhage. On the contrary, they were eager to stress the small number who had died from stroke, implying that there was no cause for concern, and absolutely no reason to stop the cholesterol campaign. The risk of dying from cerebral hemorrhage was limited, the MRFIT researchers wrote. However, calculated in the same way as is usual for CHD, the risk for individuals with low cholesterol of dying from a cerebral hemorrhage was 500 percent higher than for individuals with high cholesterol.

In the MRFIT study, only middle-aged men were studied. In this age group cerebral hemorrhage is uncommon, and the number of strokes assumed to be induced by low cholesterol may therefore be greatly underestimated. But the risk of a cerebral hemorrhage becomes more and more common with increasing age. Diet-heart proponents say that cholesterol-lowering measures are a good idea for all age groups. But we are entitled to ask whether it is, in fact, harmless to lower cholesterol in elderly people. You may remember from Chapter 6 that since the study of Blankenhorn and his associates, 190 mg/dl has been considered the lower limit for drug treatment in the US. Starting at that level and using modern cholesterol-lowering drugs in combination with diet, it is not too difficult to lower cholesterol to a level where the risk of stroke may be increased. Perhaps we should take steps to raise the blood cholesterol in older people rather than lower it.

You can guess for yourself whether the subject of increased risk of stroke or other side effects was discussed in the MRFIT report.

Maybe you will object that statin treatment *lowers* the risk of stroke. That is partially correct because stroke may be due either to a clot or thrombosis in an artery of the neck or the brain, or to a rupture of a cerebral vessel followed by a hemorrhage in the brain. And it is only the latter type of stroke that has been associated with low cholesterol.

But even if statin treatment could prevent cerebral hemorrhage, we know by now that it is not due to a lowering of cholesterol. Perhaps the statins may prevent stroke (and heart attacks) *in spite of* their effects on blood cholesterol? Perhaps the other effects of the statins outnumber the effect of low cholesterol? Or perhaps low cholesterol is only a risk marker, secondary to the real cause, just as is the case with a high cholesterol?

If you think that the potential risks connected with cholesterol-lowering have dampened the enthusiasm of those who are eager to treat the whole population, you are wrong, as you will see in the next chapter.

Myth 8

The Cholesterol Campaign is Based on Good Science

. . . the fourth and last wrong measure of probability I shall take notice of, and which keeps in ignorance or error more people than all the other together, is. . . the giving up our assent to the common received opinions, either of our friends or party, neighbourhood or country. How many men have no other ground for their tenets than the supposed honesty, or learning, or number of those of the same profession? As if honest or bookish men could not err, or truth were to be established by the vote of the multitude; yet this with most men serves the turn. If we could but see the secret motives that influenced the men of name and learning in the world, we should not always find that it was the embracing of truth for its own sake, that made them espouse the doctrines they owned, and maintained.

John Locke (1632-1704)

When two people share responsibility each will carry, at most, one percent of the burden.

Piet Hein
(1906-1996; Danish poet and physicist)

The proofs

"It has been established beyond a reasonable doubt that lowering definitely elevated blood cholesterol levels. . . will reduce the risk of heart attacks caused by coronary heart disease."

If you have read this book, you may wonder whether this statement is a drug advertisement, and if the drug company was sued for misleading advertising. The quote, however, comes word for word from the summary of the consensus conference held at the National Institutes of Health in 1984,[1] long before the introduction of the statins. The aim of this conference was to discuss how the results of the Lipid Research Clinics trial should be translated into general recommendations for the American people.

The conference was headed by Basil Rifkind, who had been the director of the trial. Professor Rifkind also determined who would be invited to join the panel that formulated the final recommendations.

Consensus in Latin means "accord" or "unanimity." But there was no accord and no unanimity among the participants. Among the many critical voices, Professor Michael Oliver from Scotland, director of the early WHO trial, stressed that the trend toward an increased mortality from other causes was as strong as the trend toward a reduced mortality from coronary heart disease. "Why explain these results away?" he asked.

A British epidemiologist named Richard Peto admitted that in every trial "something ridiculous" had happened. But, he said, while no single trial was convincing, the trial evidence was impressive when analyzed together. (Does this sound familiar?)

Biostatistician Paul Meier from the University of Chicago opposed Rifkind's description of the LRC trial. He remarked: "To call 'conclusive' a study which showed no difference in total mortality, and by the usual statistical criteria, an entirely nonsignificant difference in coronary incidents, seems to me a substantial misuse of the term."

There was no unanimity, either, about the treatment that the conference planned to recommend. One speaker at the conference advised lowering dietary cholesterol, another advised lowering dietary fat of animal origin and did not think that dietary cholesterol had any importance, a third member recommended lowering the caloric intake, no matter how.

The final statement from the conference resolved the disagreements by recommending all three dietary measures. Criticism from the audience was simply swept under the rug. Some of the critics were cut off by the panel chairman, Daniel Steinberg, who cited a lack of time. Requests to write a minority report were denied as inconsistent with the conference goal of consensus.[2]

Let us now look at the findings the panel claimed as scientific support for their recommendations. Here they are at last, all the proofs that, when added to each other, supposedly provide overwhelming support for the diet-heart idea. Knowing the radical measures that followed, we can be confident that the panel members included all available arguments. Here they come, all the strong proofs.

"Proof" number one

The inherited disorders prove that high blood cholesterol by itself can induce coronary heart disease.

This is pure speculation. What we do know is that people with inherited disorders have high cholesterol because the passage of cholesterol from blood to cell is slowed down. What we also know is that atherosclerosis is more widespread and more severe in these individuals. But is it true atherosclerosis? And is it really caused by their high cholesterol?

The peculiarities of individuals with familial hypercholesterolemia is best seen in the rare homozygous form, the form that appears when both parents have the deficient gene for the LDL-receptor. (See page 94.) Autopsy studies of such individuals show that cholesterol deposition is increased, not only in their vessels, but generally throughout their bodies. Many other organs are impregnated with cholesterol, just as we find in cholesterol-fed rabbits.

The vascular changes seen in people with the more common heterozygous form of familial hypercholesterolemia are more difficult to analyze because these changes must partially be due to the metabolic error and partly to common atherosclerosis. And how do we know whether the possible effects of treatment stem from reduction of the changes caused by the inborn error or from reduction of atherosclerosis? Thus, any conclusion that may be true for individuals with familial hypercholesterolemia cannot possibly be valid for the rest of mankind.

Besides, more recent studies that have included only or mostly patients with familial hypercholesterolemia have shown that even large reductions of their cholesterol levels are not followed by a reduction in their vascular obstructions. In other words, the changes in their coronary atherosclerosis are independent of the changes of their blood cholesterol.

"Proof" number two

Animals become atherosclerotic when they are fed diets that raise their blood cholesterol, and the atherosclerosis disappears when their cholesterol is lowered again with diet or drugs.

In Chapter 5 we saw what the animal experiments are worth as evidence. The fact that vascular changes produced by an extremely unnatural diet disappear when the diet is terminated cannot prove anything about human atherosclerosis. (Weird John's gastric ulcer, caused by swallowing iron nails, disappeared when he ceased eating hardware. But this is no proof that other patients' gastric ulcers are caused by eating building materials.)

The consensus conference report did not mention anything about experimental coronary heart disease, most likely because it is not possible to produce this disease in animals merely by increasing blood cholesterol.

"Proof" number three

There is a direct connection between blood cholesterol and the occurrence of coronary heart disease in various populations.

Look at Figures 2A, 2B, 2C and, in particular, 2D and judge for yourself.

"Proof" number four

People who have immigrated to another country with a higher average blood cholesterol level gradually acquire the dietary habits, blood cholesterol concentrations and CHD rates of their new country of residence.

The Masai, the Polynesians and many more populations that contradict this assertion were ignored, nor was anything said about Marmot's studies of the Japanese immigrants.

"Proof" number five

Severity and frequency of raised plaques in the aorta and coronary arteries are strongly correlated with blood cholesterol levels.

Amazing, isn't it? Maintain any delusion again and again, no matter how far from reality it may be, and it may finally be taken for the truth. See Chapter 4 for the facts.

"Proof" number six

Populations experiencing severe dietary (especially fat) limitations and weight loss have been shown to have less atherosclerosis and CHD and fewer heart attacks.

Many other factors besides lack of dietary fat are different in severely deprived people; no conclusions can be drawn from such observations.

"Proof" number seven

Epidemiological studies have shown that elevated blood cholesterol levels in healthy people predict the future occurrence of coronary heart disease.

. . . except for Maoris, Stockholmers, Greeks, Finns, Russians, Canadians, women, men after age 47, and for those who already have had a heart attack. (See Chapter 2.)

"Proof" number eight

Evidence emerging from multiple clinical trials clearly indicates that lowering blood cholesterol levels in patients with high blood cholesterol levels decreases the likelihood of fatal and non-fatal coronary heart disease.

A few lines after the above statement, the consensus report said that none of the previous dietary trials had proven that a lowering of blood cholesterol could diminish the incidence of coronary heart disease. In both the "proving" trials (LRC and CLAS), cholesterol had been lowered with drugs because diet was considered insufficient. Thus, the panel admitted that no trial with diet had proven beneficial and, at that time, no drug trial had lowered fatal CHD significantly.

"Proof" number nine

Thus, the evidence obtained from genetic, experimental, epidemiological and clinical intervention investigations overwhelmingly supports a causal relationship between blood cholesterol levels and coronary heart disease.

This was all of it. This is the scientific foundation for the cholesterol campaign, the numerous proofs that do not suffice one by one but that, taken together, are so "overwhelming."

The panel considered the conclusive power so great that they had no doubts when it came to recommendations.

Recommendation number one

More than a dozen randomized trials of the effects of fat-controlled diets or drugs permit the conclusion that reduction of blood cholesterol levels in people with relatively high initial levels will reduce the rate of coronary heart disease. This has been shown most convincingly in men with a high cholesterol level, but although direct intervention studies have not been conducted in women, there is no reason to propose a separate treatment schedule for women.

Nothing was said about the fact that most trials did not demonstrate *any* benefit for women—in fact, both the number of deaths and the number of heart attacks had increased in some of them; or that in most studies high cholesterol has not been associated with an increased coronary mortality for women.

Recommendation number two

Individuals in the high-risk group (above 242 mg/dl at an age of 30-39 and above 261 mg/dl at an age above 40) should primarily have intensive dietary treatment requiring a major effort on the part of physicians, nutritionists, dietitians and other health professionals. If this treatment does not work, drug therapy should be used.

Thus, in the United States alone, tens of millions of healthy individuals are to be put on a diet that is not only difficult and unsatisfying, but also dangerous. Let's hope there are enough health professionals to carry out this daring project.

The drug producers and their stockholders should be happy because, as you now know, it is extremely difficult to lower blood cholesterol with diet alone. The panel also knew it: after all, the control individuals in the LRC trial had eaten the recommended diet, and their cholesterol decreased less than one percent. No doubt about it, drugs would be necessary.

Recommendation number three

Individuals with moderate-risk blood cholesterol (above 220 mg/dl at an age of 30-39; above 240 mg/dl at an age above 40— the upper 25 percent on the cholesterol scale) should also have intensive dietary treatment, and, if other risk factors were present, drug therapy should be considered.

Further tens of millions of Americans on a drab diet and dangerous drugs! In the LRC trial only those from the upper 0.8

percent on the cholesterol scale were treated, and treated with both diet and drugs. And only after enormous effort could the trial directors come up with a result that nobody but a statistical incompetent could see as positive.

If it is that difficult with drugs to improve the prognosis for people with the most extreme cholesterol levels, how can diet alone produce a benefit for those with no more than moderately high cholesterol?

Recommendation number four

Blood cholesterol is too high in most Americans because they eat too much saturated fat, too many calories and too much cholesterol.

To avoid conflicts between the proponents, the recommendations included *all* the suggested diets.

Recommendation number five

Therefore, all Americans except children below the age of two are recommended a diet with no more than 250-300 mg cholesterol per day, and a reduction of total saturated fat intake to 10% or less of total calories, and an increase of polyunsaturated fat intake but to no more than 10% of total calories. The goal is to reduce blood cholesterol in the entire population to less than 195 mg/dl.

Here everybody is urged to eat what was originally advised for the high-risk group, except that people with normal cholesterol do not get help from health professionals. These people (the majority) have to judge for themselves when the magical 10 percent limit for polyunsaturated fat has been reached, the limit between harmless and dangerous amounts. Nobody knows how panel members arrived at the upper 10 percent limit for polyunsaturates nor why they chose a cholesterol limit of 195 mg/dl. (Every "authority" seems to have his own limit; the chosen value was probably determined by a vote.)

Recommendation number six

There is no direct evidence of the benefit to be expected in the elderly, but dietary treatment may still be helpful.

Apart from the fact that there is no evidence either for the rest of mankind, why should we sour the lives of the elderly with an unpleasant diet if its benefit has never been proven? And remember, you belong to the elderly as soon as you reach the age of 47 years.

Recommendation number seven

Also children should have treatment but not before the age of two. If blood cholesterol is above 172 mg/dl, diet is recommended; if it is above 203 mg/dl, drugs should be given, for instance, cholestyramine.

Poor kids! Remember that two out of three trial subjects who received cholestyramine had gas, heartburn, belching, bloating, abdominal pain, nausea, vomiting, constipation or diarrhea.

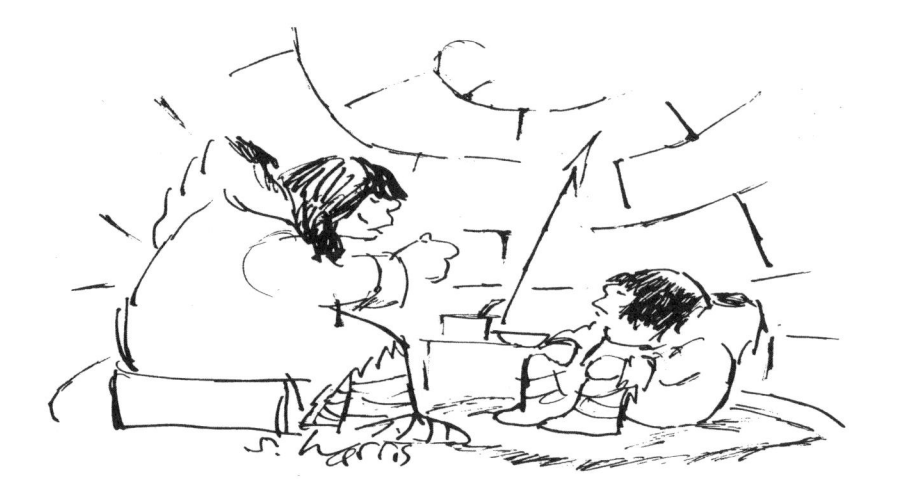

"Every day you should eat something from each of the
five basic food groups: Fried blubber, boiled blubber,
stewed blubber, baked blubber and raw blubber."

Recommendation number eight

If the American population follows the recommendations of the National Cholesterol Education Program, substantial improvements are in sight. For instance, if the cholesterol is lowered by 5 percent, the risk of having a heart attack will be reduced by 10 percent.

These figures, which are cited in all official papers on cholesterol and diet, are grossly misleading. The risk of having a heart attack in the LRC trial was lowered from 9.8 to 8.1 percent, a difference of only 1.7 percent. This equals 0.2 percentage point for each percent of cholesterol lowering, which means a total of only one percentage point if blood cholesterol is lowered by 5 percent. But this whole line of reasoning is absurd because, after all, the LRC trial did not lower the number of heart attacks more than could be explained by chance.

Recommendation number nine

The absolute magnitude of this benefit should be greater in patients at high risk from existing coronary heart disease or the presence of other risk factors such as cigarette smoking and hypertension.

This statement is preposterous. The calculations mentioned above were based on the figures from the LRC trial, which studied no one but high risk individuals.

No reservations

The panel had no reservations about these recommendations except to say that a number of problems should be investigated in the future (thus ensuring huge amounts of future government welfare for scientists and research doctors). They suggested, for instance, that more information should be gained about the possible danger of eating large amounts of polyunsaturated oil. Let us hope that a diet very high in polyunsaturated fatty acids is not harmful, but it would have been wise to perform such studies before launching a campaign to change the way mankind has eaten for thousands of years.

The recommendations of the National Cholesterol Education Campaign prompted protests from many scientists[3] but, as we know, without any impact whatsoever. The cholesterol campaign has flourished ever since and has spread to many other countries. Rumors are circulating that Ancel Keys has been suggested as a candidate for the Nobel prize.

Nothing was mentioned in the consensus report about the numerous unsupportive studies I have discussed in this book. And contrary to the initial statement of the consensus report, scientists are *not* in agreement about the dangers of high-fat food and cholesterol. In the next chapter, I shall present some of the critics and their objections.

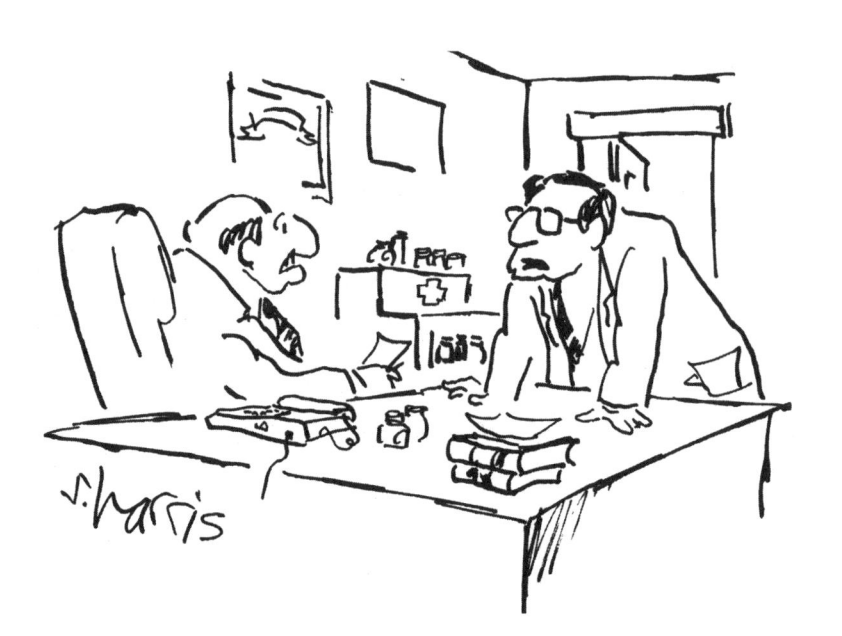

"You must realize, Erskin, that preventive medicine does not consist in giving patients medication for diseases they don't have."

© 2000 by Sidney Harris

CHOLESTEROL LOWERING IN CHILDREN

Zealous proponents of the cholesterol hypothesis argue that we should begin cholesterol-lowering measures in childhood. They say that atherosclerosis starts in the early years; therefore, all parents should test their children's cholesterol and teach them to eat "properly," beginning at the age of two. This age limit was chosen because, in spite of their clever persuasions, diet-heart proponents would have difficulty convincing parents that whole milk, an allegedly poisonous food for adults, is harmful to babies. So "intervention" is held off until the tender age of 24 months, when most youngsters in the US are put on skimmed milk, milk substitutes and low-fat foods.

The argument for giving growing children a draconian diet can be made by claiming that the fatty streaks, the thin layer of cholesterol-laden cells situated on the inside of most arteries, are the forerunners of atherosclerosis. These fatty streaks appear even before we are born and are found in the vessels of all children, even in populations where atherosclerosis is rare. The public has not been told that the presence of fatty streaks does not mean that atherosclerosis will develop, and that there is no evidence that these fatty streaks are due to high cholesterol, or that they will disappear if we lower cholesterol in children.

In addition, high cholesterol in childhood does not mean that cholesterol will be high later in life. Several studies have shown that about half the children with high cholesterol at age two have normal cholesterol when they reach puberty.

And even if high cholesterol in childhood remained high in adulthood and predicted cardiovascular disease later in life, how should we treat the children? The answer from the proponents is: by diet! For this reason, many children are now being fed chemically processed margarine and a variety of processed, synthetic, low-fat products instead of nutritious and natural foods like whole milk, cheese, meat and eggs.

And the effect of diet on blood cholesterol is hardly measurable, especially in children. The only way to lower cholesterol effectively is by drugs—even the proponents admit that. But even if we had evidence that cholesterol-lowering measures begun at the age of two were of benefit, we have no evidence that these measures would compensate for the side effects of an unhealthy diet or daily intake of drugs for many years because, luckily, such trials have never been carried out.

At best, emphasis on lowering cholesterol in children will create families of unhappy hypochondriacs, obsessed with their diet and blood chemistry. At worst, it will have profound and unfortunate effects on the growth of children because foods containing cholesterol and animal fats are rich in important nutrients.

Ravnskov U. Prevention of atherosclerosis in children. *The Lancet* 355, 69, 2000.

Myth 9

All Scientists Support the Diet-Heart Idea

Only dead fishes go downstream.
                                    Polish proverb

At this point many readers are probably wondering why they have not heard about all this before.

Criticism has been raised—a great deal of criticism. But it has been presented in journals and books that are not easily accessible to the layman, and critical voices have been drowned out in a flood of papers from the proponents. And the media, supported in large part by advertising revenues from pharmaceuticals and a food industry that has found it extremely profitable to use vegetable oils, has consistently ignored the voices of dissent while hyping the recommendations for expensive drugs and dietary change.

Presented here, in alphabetic order, are a few of the scientists who have had the courage to swim against the current. All of them have produced a large number of scientific studies of which I shall mention only the most important.

Mary Enig

Dr. Enig is an international expert in the field of lipid biochemistry, a nutritionist and a consulting editor to a number of scientific publications, including the *Journal of the American College of Nutrition*. She is also President of the Maryland Nutritionists Association. Her main research has concerned the hazards associated with consumption of *trans* fatty acids.[1] She has published many scientific papers on the subject of food, nutrition, food fats and oils; several chapters on nutrition for text books; and a primer for laymen and professionals on fats, oils and cholesterol.[2] When asked whether saturated fats cause heart disease, she replied:

The idea that saturated fats cause heart disease is completely wrong, but the statement has been "published" so many times over the last three or more decades that it is very difficult to convince people otherwise unless they are willing to take the time to read and learn what all the economic and political factors were that produced the anti-saturated-fat agenda.

Michael Gurr

Dr. Gurr is an associate professor of biochemistry at the School of Biological & Molecular Sciences in Oxford, editor-in-chief of *Nutrition Research Reviews* and editor of three other scientific journals. In a recent 50-page review published in *Progress in Lipid Research,* he presented the arguments of the cholesterol hypothesis in a thorough and honest way along with all the weaknesses of the theory.[3] His main objections were the insufficient correspondence in vascular pathology between animal models and man and between familial hypercholesterolemia and atherosclerosis; the flaws and selection bias in the epidemiological evidence; the lack of correspondence between trends in coronary mortality and fat consumption; the weak prediction that can be achieved by measuring blood cholesterol; and the lack of improvement in mortality after dietary and pharmacological lowering of blood cholesterol. Professor Gurr's final words provide a fitting summary of everything that we have discussed in this book:

The arguments and discussion of the scientific evidence presented in this review will not convince those "experts" who have already made up their minds, for whatever reason, be it truly scientific or political, that a fatty diet is the cause of CHD. How-

ever, I hope that some readers, who were, perhaps, unaware that the lipid hypothesis had any shortcomings, will have been persuaded that the relationships between the fats we eat and the likelihood that we may die from a heart attack is by no means as simple as these simplistic statements imply.

George Mann

Now retired, Professor Mann was previously a professor in medicine and biochemistry at Vanderbilt University in Tennessee. From his studies of the Masai, he realized that animal fat could not possibly be the main cause of high cholesterol and coronary heart disease. As long ago as 1977, in the *New England Journal of Medicine,* he presented his main arguments against the diet-heart idea: the lack of relationship between dietary habits and blood cholesterol, the lack of correlation between this century's trends in fat consumption and death rates in the United States, and the disappointing outcome of the cholesterol-lowering trials.[4]

Eight years later, when the cholesterol education campaign was getting into gear, Professor Mann summarized his criticism of the diet-heart idea in *Nutrition Today.*[5] The diet-heart idea is the greatest scientific deception of our times, he said. Mann is especially critical of the cholesterol-lowering trials. Never in the history of science have so many costly experiments failed so consistently, he declared.

Professor Mann severely criticized the LRC directors. The unsupportive results from the LRC study have not prevented them from "bragging about this cataclysmic breakthrough," he wrote. And he continued:

The managers at the National Institutes of Health have used Madison Avenue hype to sell this failed trial in the way the media people sell an underarm deodorant. The Bethesda Consensus Panel. . . has failed to acknowledge that the LRC trial, like so many before it, is saying firmly and loudly: "No, the diet you used is not an effective way to manage cholesterolemia or prevent coronary heart disease and the drug you so generously tested for a pharmaceutical house does not work either."

People who are faced with the many distorted facts about diet, cholesterol and heart disease often ask me why almost all scientists unquestioningly accept the diet-heart idea. And you may have asked the same question after reading this book. Here is Professor Mann's comment:

Fearing to loose their soft money funding, the academicians who should speak up and stop this wasteful anti-science are strangely quiet. Their silence has delayed a solution for coronary heart disease by a generation.

Professor Mann offers a little glimpse of hope at the end of his article in *Nutrition Today*:

Those who manipulate data do not appreciate that understanding the nature of things cannot be permanently distorted— the true explanations cannot be permanently ignored. Inexorably, truth is revealed and deception is exposed. . . In due time truth will come out. This is the relieving grace in this sorry sequence.

Michael F. Oliver

A former professor and director of the Wynn Institute for Metabolic Research, London, Professor Oliver was one of the first to demonstrate that, on average, patients with coronary heart disease were more likely to have abnormal levels of various fats in the blood than did control individuals. Professor Oliver still thinks that selected groups of patients, mostly those with inherited diseases of cholesterol metabolism, may benefit from cholesterol lowering, but in several papers he has warned against campaigns for cholesterol lowering in the general population. For example, he has written:

Doubts about the promotional nature of these campaigns are not popular. Doubters are scorned, although this does not matter. But the issue is a very serious one if vast sums are spent and widespread changes are made in the life-style of normal people when the accumulated evidence is that total mortality is unchanged or possibly even increased.[6]

Again and again, Oliver has criticized those who think that the increased mortality from nonmedical causes seen in many trials is an effect of chance. Rather, he thinks, the very reduction of blood cholesterol may be dangerous because of unforeseen long-term effects on the composition of cell membranes.[7] According to Professor Oliver, our bodies may regulate attempts to lower blood cholesterol in most cases, but

. . . would such homoeostatic [regulatory] mechanisms be effective in all patients, at all times, and in all cells—particularly cells in which biologic function is impaired for other reasons? These doubts will not go away for several more years.[6]

Professor Oliver also feels uneasy about the relationship between low cholesterol and cancer.

It should be mentioned, however, that after the publication of the recent statin trials, Professor Oliver changed his mind and now says that cholesterol should be lowered, but only for patients at very high risk.

Edward R. Pinckney

Dr. Pinckney was an editor of four medical journals and former co-editor of the *Journal of the American Medical Association.* In 1973, he published a book called *The Cholesterol Controversy,* which summarized all the inconsistencies in the cholesterol idea.[8] It seems impossible that any sensible and honest doctor who has read this book could continue to teach his patients about the dangers of cholesterol.

Dr. Pinckney describes all the factors that influence blood cholesterol in healthy people and how difficult it is to get a reliable measure of the cholesterol level due to uncertainties of the analysis:

The level of one's blood cholesterol is, at best, nothing more than an extremely rough indication of a great many different disease conditions. At worst, it can be more the cause of stress and the diseases that stress brings on. To alter one's life-style as a consequence of this particular laboratory test may well cause more trouble than it could relieve.

Dr. Pinckney thoroughly describes the dangers of lowering one's cholesterol and devotes an entire chapter to the political drama preceding the cholesterol campaign. Pinckney had long wondered about the dairy industry's passive acceptance of the slurs against its products. The explanation he found was that many dairy distributors also distributed polyunsaturated products at an even greater profit. And the dairy farmer does not protest because the federal government uses taxpayer money to buy the farmer's surplus butter at a price far higher than what he could make by competing on the open market.

The beginning of Chapter 1 in Dr. Pinckney's book is worth citing:

Your fear of dying—if you happen to be one of the great many people who suffer from this morbid preoccupation—may well have made you a victim of the cholesterol controversy. For, if you have come to believe that you can ward off death from heart disease by altering the amount of cholesterol in your blood, whether by diet or by drugs, you are following a regime that still has no basis in fact. Rather, you as a consumer have been taken in by certain commercial interests and health groups who are more interested in your money than your life.

Raymond Reiser

Dr. Reiser is a former professor of biochemistry at Texas A & M University. In 1973 he criticized the recommendations for dietary treatment of high cholesterol by declaring:

The authority quoted by these authors for the recommendation is not a primary source but another review similar to their own. It is this practice of referring to secondary or tertiary sources, each taking the last on faith, which has led to the matter-of-fact acceptance of a phenomenon that may not exist.

Unfortunately, Professor Reiser's words have not had any

influence, as you may recall from the section on "good" and "bad" cholesterol in Chapter 2. In his paper, Professor Reiser continued with a thorough 30-page review of almost all experiments on the influence of dietary fatty acids on blood cholesterol levels. His main conclusions were that most experiments are biased by serious faults, that limited time frames and too few test individuals have been used, and that the diet studied has been too extreme to allow conclusions that are valid for ordinary people. Furthermore, some saturated fatty acids have no influence on the blood cholesterol level at all, while others may raise it, but not to high levels. Professor Reiser therefore stated:

One must be bold indeed to attempt to persuade large segments of the populations of the world to change their accustomed diets and to threaten important branches of agriculture and agribusiness with the results of such uncontrolled, primitive, trial-and-error type explorations. Certainly modern science is capable of better research when so much is at stake.[9]

More recently, Professor Reiser analyzed the references used as support by the American Heart Association in its rationale for its dietary recommendations. He could not find any supportive studies. In fact, some of the studies had results that contradicted the diet-heart idea:

Thus the rationale is not a logical explanation of the dietary recommendations but an assemblage of obsolete and misquoted references. Since rational explanations for the recommendations are essential for their acceptance, the public to whom they are addressed is justified in remaining skeptical of them.[10]

Paul Rosch

Dr. Paul J. Rosch is President of the American Institute of Stress, Clinical Professor of Medicine and Psychiatry at New York Medical College, Honorary Vice President of the International Stress Management Association and Chairman of its US branch. He is the editor or subeditor of three well-known medical journals, he has been a member of the board of several other journals. He has served as President of the New York State Society of Internal Medicine, as Chairman of the International Foundation for Biopsychosocial Development and Human Health and has been an Expert Consultant on Stress to the United States Centers for Disease Control. He has written extensively over the past forty-five years on the role of stress in health and illness, with particular reference to cardiovascular disease and cancer. He has appeared on numerous national and international television programs such as *The Today Show*, *Good Morning America*, *60 Minutes*, *Nova* and on CBS, NBC, PBS, BBC and CBC network presentations. His editorials and comments have been published in every major medical journal. Professor Rosch has also been interviewed and widely quoted in numerous major American newspapers and magazines.

As the author of the *Newsletter of the American Institute of Stress*, Professor Rosch has published several articles about the cholesterol hypothesis and the diet-heart idea. His conclusions

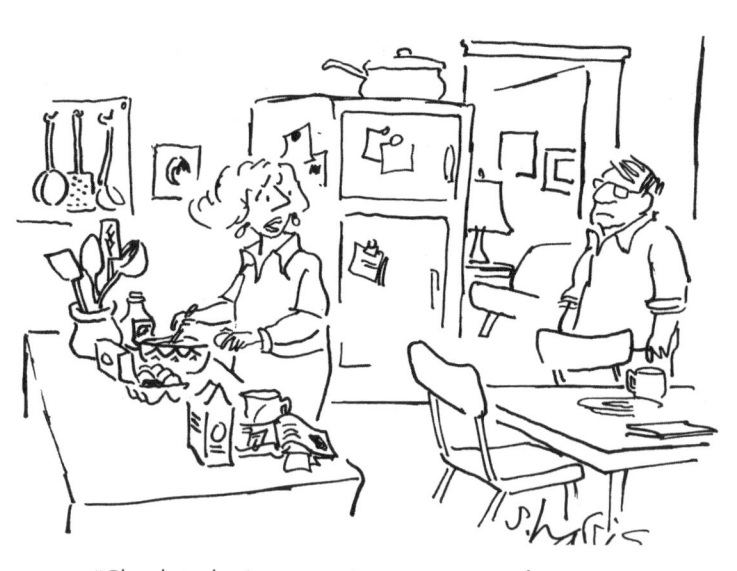

"Check today's paper. Are eggs now safe to eat,
or should we continue to avoid them like the plague?""

are close to those presented in this book: *A massive crusade has been conceived to "lower your cholesterol count" by rigidly restricting dietary fat, coupled with aggressive drug treatment. Much of the impetus for this comes from speculation, rather than any solid scientific proof.*

The result is well-known, says Professor Rosch: *The public is so brainwashed, that many people believe that the lower your cholesterol, the healthier you will be or the longer you will live. Nothing could be further from the truth.*

How can this go on year after year? Professor Rosch has several explanations: *The cholesterol cartel of drug companies, manufacturers of low-fat foods, blood-testing devices and others with huge vested financial interests have waged a highly successful promotional campaign. Their power is so great that they have infiltrated medical and governmental regulatory agencies that would normally protect us from such unsubstantiated dogma.*

Professor Rosch reminds us that practicing physicians get most of their information from the drug companies. But, *compared to their peers a half century ago, most doctors don't have the time or skills to critically evaluate reports, very few know anything about research, nor did the generation that taught them.*[11]

Ray Rosenman

Dr. Rosenman is the retired Director of Cardiovascular Research in the Health Sciences Program at SRI International in Menlo Park, California, and Associate Chief of Medicine, Mt. Zion Hospital and Medical Center in San Francisco. He has been a cardiologist and a researcher since 1950. He has published four books, many textbook chapters and numerous journal articles about cardiovascular diseases. His main interest has been the influence of neurogenic and psychological factors on the blood lipids, but he has also written reviews critical of the diet-heart idea.[12] Here is the conclusion from his most recent review:

These data lead to a conclusion that neither diet, serum lipids, nor their changes can explain wide national and regional differences of IHD [coronary heart disease] rates, nor the variable 20th century rises and declines of CHD mortality.

This conclusion is supported by the results of many clinical trials which fail to provide adequate evidence that lowering serum cholesterol, particularly by dietary changes, is associated with a significant reduction of IHD mortality or improved longevity. It is variously stated that the preventive effects of dietary and drug treatments have been exaggerated by a tendency in trial reports, reviews, and other papers to cite and inflate supportive results, while suppressing discordant data, and many such examples are cited.

Russell Smith

The late Dr. Smith was an American experimental psychologist with a strong background in physiology, mathematics and engineering. In cooperation with Edward Pinckney, he studied all aspects of the diet-cholesterol-heart issue with extreme thoroughness and presented his findings in two large scientific reviews of the literature[13] containing more than 700 pages with more than 3000 references, as well as in a popular book.[14] No review written by the proponents of the diet-heart idea can compare with Russell Smith's books when it comes to completeness and scientific depth. Volume 1 of his review is an overview of the entire issue. Smith's summation is devastating for the diet-heart proponents:

Although the public generally perceives medical research as the highest order of precision, much of the epidemiologic research is, in fact, rather imprecise and understandably so because it has been conducted principally by individuals with no formal education and little on-the-job training in the scientific method. Consequently, studies are often poorly designed and data are often inappropriately analyzed and interpreted. Moreover, biases are so commonplace, they appear to be the rule, rather than the exception. It is virtually impossible not to recognize that many researchers routinely manipulate and/or interpret their data to fit preconceived hypotheses, rather than manipulate hypotheses to fit their data. Much of the literature, therefore, is nothing less than an affront to the discipline of science.

Russell Smith concludes:

The current campaign to convince every American to change his or her diet and, in many cases, to initiate drug "therapy" for life is based on fabrications, erroneous interpretations and/or gross exaggerations of findings and, very importantly, the ignoring of massive amounts of unsupportive data. . . It does not seem possible that objective scientists without vested interests could ever interpret the literature as supportive.

In his books and papers Russell Smith criticizes a large number of leading scientists from the National Heart, Lung and Blood Institute and the American Heart Association, which he calls the "alliance." He considers their work "incompetent and sloppy."

The fraud is so blatant and so pervasive that it was considered necessary to take some liberties with the usual staid rhetoric of a scientific review and inject stronger language to emphasize the problem.

Russell Smith is aware that he is up against some extremely powerful institutions:

The political and financial power of the NHLBI and AHA team. . . is enormous and without equal. And because the alliance has substantial credibility in the eyes of the public and most practicing physicians, it has become a juggernaut, able to use its power and prestige to suppress a great body of unsupportive evidence and even defy the most fundamental tool of scientists, logic.

The scientists who have produced the misleading papers and reviews are, of course, the first with whom Russell Smith finds fault. But he adds:

Equally culpable are the editors of the many journals who

*publish articles without regard to their quality or scientific im-
port. It is depressing to know that billions of dollars and a highly
sophisticated medical research system are being wasted chasing
windmills.*

William E. Stehbens

Another articulate critic, Dr. Stehbens is a professor at the
Department of Pathology, Wellington School of Medicine, and director of the Malaghan Institute of Medical Research in Wellington, New Zealand. Based on his own studies and on extensive
reviews of the literature, he has effectively demonstrated the many
fallacies of the diet-heart idea. In a thorough review of the experimental studies he concluded:

*Upon examination of this evidence and consideration of the
specific criteria for the experimental production of atherosclerosis, any pathologist of independent mind and free from preconceived ideas would conclude that human atherosclerosis and
the lesions induced by the dietary overload of cholesterol and
fats are not one and the same disease.*

Professor Stehbens has also pointed out the weaknesses of
the epidemiological studies that have used mortality statistics as
proof for causality:

*Continued, unquestioned use of unreliable data has led to
premature conclusions and the sacrifice of truth. The degree of
inaccuracy of vital statistics for CHD is of such uncertain magnitude that, when superimposed on other deficiencies already indicated, the concept of an epidemic rise and decline of CHD in
many countries must be regarded as unproven, and governmental or health policies based on unreliable data become completely
untenable.*

According to Stehbens, atherosclerosis is due to wear and
tear of the arteries, and not to high cholesterol levels in the blood,
an idea he supports with many good arguments.[15] (See the Introduction.)

The following words from a 1988 paper summarize

Stehbens' view on the diet-heart idea:

The perpetuation of the cholesterol myth and the alleged preventive measures are doing the dairy and meat industries of this and other countries much harm quite apart from their potential to endanger optimum nutrition levels and the health of the populace at large. . . It is essential to adhere to hard scientific facts and logic. Scientific evidence for the role of dietary fat and hypercholesterolemia in the causation of atherosclerosis is seriously lacking. . . The lipid hypothesis has enjoyed undeserved longevity and respectability. Readers should be aware of the unscientific nature of claims used to support it and see it as little more than a pernicious bum steer.

Lars Werkö

Now retired, Professor Werkö was previously a professor of medicine at Sahlgren's Hospital, Gothenburg, Sweden, scientific director at the Astra Company, and then head of the Swedish Council on Technology Assessment in Health Care, a governmental agency. Professor Werkö has been an opponent of the diet-heart idea for many years. In 1976 he criticized the design of the large epidemiological studies aimed at preventing coronary heart disease, most of all the Framingham study.

According to Werkö, the dogma is based on questionable "facts" rooted in hopes, wishful thinking and studies using selected materials.[16]

No studies have proved anything, but instead of formulating new hypotheses, diet-heart supporters call the current one the most probable truth, and they have intervened in people's lives because they will not wait for the final proof.

In a recent paper, he pointed to a number of inaccuracies and sloppy data gathering in the MRFIT trial. (See page 50.)

These are only some of the many critics of the diet-heart idea. In the reference section you will find many more.[17]

Epilogue

After a lecture, a journalist asked me how she could be certain that my information was not just as biased as that of the cholesterol campaign. At first I did not know what to say. Afterwards I found the answer.

She could not be certain. Everyone must gain the truth in an active way. If you want to know something you must look at all the premises yourself, listen to all the arguments yourself, and then decide for yourself what seems to be the most likely answer. You may be easily led astray if you ask the authorities to do this work for you.

This is also the answer to those who wonder why even honest scientists are misled. And it is also the answer to those who, after reading this book, ask the same question.

References

Introduction

1. Olsson B. Hur upplevs deltagande i riskfaktor screaning? *Allmän Medicin* 11, 144-147, 1990.
2. Stehbens WE. The lipid hypothesis and the role of hemodynamics in atherogenesis. *Progress in Cardiovascular Diseases* 33, 119-136, 1990.
3. The idea that the extra-arterial pressure is important for the development of atherosclerosis comes from Saul GD, Gerard, HM. Physical fitness, dynamic extra-arterial pressures, and the pathogenesis and distribution of atherosclerosis. *Medical Hypotheses* 36, 228-237, 1991, and Saul GD. Arterial stress from intraluminal pressure modified by tissue pressure offers a complete explanation for the distribution of atherosclerosis. *Medical Hypotheses* 52, 349-351, 1999.
4. Blumgart HL, Schlesinger MJ, Davis D. Studies on the relation of the clinical manifestations of angina pectoris, coronary thrombosis and myocardial infarction to the pathological findings. *American Heart Journal* 19, 1-91, 1940.

Chapter 1

1. Keys A. Atherosclerosis: A problem in newer public health. *Journal of Mount Sinai Hospital* 20, 118-139, 1953.
2. Payer L. *Medicine & Culture.* Henry Holt & Co, New York 1988. In her book Payer describes the great differences in medical thinking and treatment in the United States, England, West Germany and France.
3. Yerushalmy J, Hilleboe HE. Fat in the diet and mortality from heart disease. A methodologic note. *The New York State Journal of Medicine* 57, 2343-2354, 1957. Although Yerushalmy and Hilleboe were critical of Keys' ideas and his use of statistics, these authors were cited by Stamler as supporters of the diet-heart idea. (Levy RI, Rifkind BM, Dennis BH, Ernst ND (edit): *Nutrition, Lipids, and Coronary Heart Disease.* A Global View. Raven Press 1979, p. 32.)
4. Kircher T, Nelson J, Burdo H. The autopsy as a measure of accuracy of the death certificate. *New England Journal of Medicine* 313, 1263-

1269, 1985; Carter JR. The problematic death certificate. *New England Journal of Medicine* 313, 1285-1286, 1985; Stehbens WE. An appraisal of the epidemic rise of coronary heart disease and its decline. *The Lancet* 1, 606-611, 1987.

5. Lundberg GD, Voigt GE. Reliability of a presumptive diagnosis in sudden unexpected deaths in adults. *Journal of the American Medical Association* 242, 2328-2330, 1979.

6. Zarling EJ, Sexton H, Milnor P. Failure to diagnose acute myocardial infarction. *Journal of the American Medical Association* 250, 1177-1181, 1983.

7. Reid DD, Rose GA. Assessing the comparability of mortality statistics. *British Medical Journal* 2, 1437-1439, 1964.

8. Wolf, S. *The Artery and the Process of Atherosclerosis* (2). Plenum Press, New York 1972, table 2, p 31.

9. Yudkin J. Diet and coronary thrombosis. Hypothesis and fact. *The Lancet* 2, 155-162, 1957.

10. Keys, A. Coronary heart disease in seven countries. *Circulation* 41, suppl. 1, 1-211, 1970.

11. However, in conflict with his figures, Keys wrote that the inhabitants in North Karelia had definitely higher cholesterol values.

12. Masironi R. Dietary factors and coronary heart disease. *Bulletin of the World Health Organization* 42, 103-114, 1970. Masironi found a connection between the consumption of fat and other dietary constituents and mortality from coronary heart disease in various countries, but also between the per capita income and coronary mortality. On the other hand, he found no parallel between the trends of fat consumption and coronary mortality. Masironi concluded that nothing proved that dietary fat played more than a marginal role in the causation of coronary heart disease. But Masironi is cited (Truswell AS. *Postgraduate Medical Journal* 52, 424-432, 1976) as a support for the diet-heart idea: "In comparisons between different communities the rate of clinical coronary heart disease correlates better with the average saturated or animal fat intake than with any other dietary index (Keys 1970; Masironi 1970)."

13. Slattery ML, Randall DE. Trends in coronary heart disease mortality and food consumption in the United States between 1909 and 1980. *American Journal of Clinical Nutrition* 47,1060-1070, 1988; Antar MA, Ohlson MA, Hogdes RE. Changes in retail market food supplies in the United States in the last seventy years in relation to the incidence of coronary heart disease, with special reference to dietary carbohydrates and essential fatty acids. *American journal of Clinical Nutrition* 14, 169-178, 1964.

14. Sytkowski PA, Kannel, WB, D'Agostino RB: Changes in risk factors and the decline in mortality from cardiovascular disease. The Framingham Heart Study. *New England Journal of Medicine* 322, 1635-41, 1990. It is not possible to see when the downward trend started, and it is a striking fact that no decline was observed for non-fatal heart attacks.

15. In the early cholesterol-lowering trials, however, the number of non-fatal heart attacks has been lowered but not the number of fatal cases. But here the authors' argument is the reverse, that it takes more time to prevent the fatal cases. More about that in Chapter 6.

16. (a) Oshima K. Statistical trend in the incidence of cerebrovascular accidents and coronary heart disease in Japan. In: Schettler G, Goto Y, Hata Y, Klose G (edit). *International symposium on atherosclerosis IV.* Springer-Verlag, Berlin 1977; (b) Kimura N. Changing patterns of coronary heart disease, stroke, and nutrient intake in Japan. *Preventive Medicine* 12, 222-227, 1983; (c) Ueshima H, Tatara K, Asakura S. Declining mortality from ischemic heart disease and changes in coronary risk factors in Japan, 1956-1980. *American Journal of Epidemiology* 125, 62-72, 1987. The authors thought that the decreasing mortality was due to better treatment of high blood pressure, but it has never been shown that lowering the blood pressure has more than a minimal effect on coronary heart disease.

17. Shimamoto T and others. Trends for coronary heart disease and stroke and their risk factors in Japan. *Circulation* 79, 503-515, 1989.

18. Guberan E. Surprising decline of cardiovascular mortality in Switzerland: 1951-1976. *Journal of Epidemiology and Community Health* 33, 114-120, 1979.

19. Mann's descriptions of the Masai tribe are found in the following papers: (a) Mann GV, Shaffer RD, Sandstead HH. Cardiovascular disease in the Masai. *Journal of Atherosclerosis Research* 4, 289-312, 1964; (b) Mann GV, Shaffer RD, Rich A. Physical fitness and immunity to heart disease in Masai. *The Lancet* 2, 1308-1310, 1965; (c) Mann GV, Shaffer R. Cholesteremia in pregnant Masai women. *Journal of the American Medical Association* 197, 123-125, 1966; (d) Mann GV, and others. Atherosclerosis in the Masai. *American Journal of Epidemiology* 95, 26-37, 1972.

20. Shaper AG. Cardiovascular studies in the Samburu tribe of northern Kenya. *American Heart Journal* 63, 437-442, 1962. Camel herdsmen in Somalia who live almost entirely on camel's milk also have very low cholesterol values: Lapiccirella V, and others. Enquete clinique, biologique et cardiographique parmi les tribus nomades de la Somalie qui se nourissent seulement de lait. *Bulletin of the World Health Organization* 27, 681-97, 1962.

21. Publishing the same result in two or more journals was fairly common years ago. It was considered an easy way for a scientific climber to improve his personal record. Today editors of medical journals disapprove of double publications; a researcher may get into serious trouble trying to publish his results in more than one journal. These are Taylor's four papers: (a) Biss K, Taylor CB, Lewis LA, Mikkelson B, Hussey LK, Ho K-J. The Masai's protection against atherosclerosis. *Pathology and Microbiology* 35, 198-204, 1970; (b) Ho K-J, Biss K, Mikkelson B, Lewis LA, Taylor CB. The Masai of East Africa: Some unique biological characteristics. *Archives of Pathology* 91, 387-410, 1971; (c) Biss K, Ho K-J, Mikkelson B, Lewis L, Taylor CB: Some unique biologic char-

acteristics of the Masai of East Africa. *New England Journal of Medicine* 284, 694-699, 1971; (d) Biss K, Taylor CB, Lewis LA, Mikkelson B, Ho K. Atherosclerosis and lipid metabolism in the Masai of East Africa. *African Journal of the Medical Sciences* 2, 249-257, 1971

22. Taylor knew how to decide whether their cholesterol metabolism was inherited or not. In the US he studied a 24-year-old Masai student and found that his cholesterol was as low as that of his comrades back in Kenya, a finding he claimed was a proof of his idea. But to use a determination from only one individual as a scientific proof is appalling, bearing in mind the great variations of blood cholesterol between different human beings.

23. Day J and others. Anthropometric, physiological and biochemical differences between urban and rural Maasai. *Atherosclerosis* 23, 357-361, 1976.

24. Keys A. Coronary heart disease - the global picture. *Atherosclerosis* 22, 149-192, 1975.

25. Charters AD, Arya BP. Incidence of ischaemic heart disease among Indians in Kenya. *The Lancet* 1, 288-289, 1960.

26. Malhotra SL, Epidemiology of ischaemic heart disease in India with special reference to causation. *British Heart Journal* 29, 895-905, 1967.

27. Zukel WJ and others. A short-term community study of the epidemiology of coronary heart disease. *American Journal of Public Health* 49, 1630-1639, 1959.

28. Finegan A and others. Diet and coronary heart disease: dietary analysis on 100 male patients. *American Journal of Clinical Nutrition* 21, 143-148, 1968.

29. Kushi LH and others. Diet and 20-year mortality from coronary heart disease. The Ireland-Boston diet-heart study. *New England Journal of Medicine* 312, 811-818, 1985.

30. Supporters of the diet-heart idea frequently refer to the Boston-Ireland study, usually in a misleading way. For instance, Zilversmit in a textbook (*Nutrition, Lipids, and Coronary Heart Disease. A Global View*. Edit. Levy RI, Rifkind BM, Dennis BH, Ernst ND. Raven Press, New York 1979, p. 159) said that coronary mortality among the Boston brothers was twice that of the two other groups. In fact, the relative risk after correction for age was 1.16 for the Boston brothers and 1.01 for the immigrant brothers compared to the Irish brothers, a statistically non-significant difference. The same author also wrote that the Irish brothers ate considerably more fiber than the Boston brothers, when, in fact, they ate less (0.64 versus 0.78 gram per 1000 calories).

31. Gordon T and others. Diet and its relation to coronary heart disease and death in three populations. *Circulation* 63, 500-515, 1981.

32. McGee DL and others. Ten-year incidence of coronary heart disease in the Honolulu heart program. Relationship to nutrient intake. *American Journal of Epidemiology* 119, 667-676, 1984.

33. Ravnskov U. The questionable role of saturated and polyunsaturated fatty acids in cardiovascular disease. *Journal of Clinical Epidemiol-*

ogy 51, 443-460, 1998.

34. National Research Council. *Diet and Health. Implications for Reducing Chronic Disease Risk.* National Academy Press, Washington, DC, 1989. The citation is found on page 193.

35. Gotto AM, LaRosa JC, Hunninghake D and others. The cholesterol facts. A summary of the evidence relating dietary fats, serum cholesterol and coronary heart disease. A joint statement by the American Heart Association and the National Heart, Lung and Blood Institute. *Circulation* 81, 1721-33, 1990. The citation is found on page 1725.

36. Paul O and others. A longitudinal study of coronary heart disease. *Circulation* 28, 20-31, 1963.

37. Kannel, WB, Gordon T. The Framingham diet study: diet and the regulation of serum cholesterol. *The Framingham study. An Epidemiologic Investigation of Cardiovascular Disease.* Section 24, Washington, DC, 1970.

38. Garcia-Palmieri MR and others. Relationship of dietary intake to subsequent coronary heart disease incidence: The Puerto Rico heart health program. *American Journal of Clinical Nutrition* 33, 1818-1827, 1980.

39. Gordon T and others. Diet and its relation to coronary heart disease and death in three populations. *Circulation* 63, 500-515, 1981.

40. McGee DL and others. Ten-year incidence of coronary heart disease in the Honolulu heart program. Relationship to nutrient intake. *American Journal of Epidemiology* 119, 667-676, 1984.

41. Kromhout D, Coulander CDL. Diet, prevalence and 10-year mortality from coronary heart disease in 871 middle-aged men. The Zutphen Study. *American Journal of Epidemiology* 119, 733-741, 1984.

42. Khaw, KT, Barrett-Connor E. Dietary fiber and reduced ischemic heart disease mortality rates in men and women: A 12-year prospective study. *American Journal of Epidemiology* 126, 1093-1102, 1987.

43. Esrey KL and others. Relationship between dietary intake and coronary heart disease mortality: Lipid Research Clinics prevalence follow-up study. *Journal of Clinical Epidemiology* 49, 211-216, 1996.

44. Bassett DR and others. Coronary heart disease in Hawaii: Dietary intake, depot fat, "stress," smoking, and energy balance in Hawaiian and Japanese men. *American Journal of Clinical Nutrition* 22, 1483-1503, 1969.

45. A recent study including more countries than in the previous ones found only a weak, positive correlation between consumption of animal fat and heart mortality. Furthermore, it found a much higher but negative correlation to other diseases, for instance, to stroke, stomach cancer and other gastro-intestinal diseases (Jacobs D and others. Report of the conference on low blood cholesterol mortality associations. *Circulation* 86, 1046-60, 1992).

46. Taubes G. Nutrition: The soft science of dietary fat. *Science Magazine* 292,2536-2545, 2001.

47. Critical letters from Scott Grundy and others were published in *Science Magazine* 2001 August 3; 293: 801-804 together with Gary Taubes' answer.

Chapter 2

1. Kannel WB. The role of cholesterol in coronary atherogenesis. *Medical Clinics of North America* 58, 363-379, 1974.

2. Stamler J, Wentworth D, Neaton JD. Is relationship between serum cholesterol and risk of premature death from coronary heart disease continuous and graded? *Journal of the American Medical Association* 256, 2823-2828, 1986.

3. To be statistically correct, deciles are not defined in this way, but as all diet-heart papers have used this definition I have used it also, to avoid confusion.

4. Kannel WB, Castelli WP, Gordon T. Cholesterol in the prediction of atherosclerotic disease. *Annals of Internal Medicine* 90, 85-91, 1979.

5. Anderson KM, Castelli WP, Levy D. Cholesterol and mortality. 30 years of follow-up from the Framingham Study. *Journal of the American Medical Association* 257, 2176-2180, 1987.

6. Simons LA and others. Risk factors for coronary heart disease in the prospective Dubbo study of Australian elderly. *Atherosclerosis* 117, 107-118, 1995.

7. Zimetbaum P and others. Plasma lipids and lipoproteins and the incidence of cardiovascular disease in the very elderly. The Bronx aging study. *Arteriosclerosis* 12, 416-423, 1992.

8. Krumholz HM and others. Lack of association between cholesterol and coronary heart disease mortality and morbidity and all-cause mortality in persons older than 70 years. *Journal of the American Medical Association* 272, 1335-1340, 1994

9. Gotto AM, LaRosa JC, Hunninghake D and others. The cholesterol facts. A summary of the evidence relating dietary fats, serum cholesterol and coronary heart disease. A joint statement by the American Heart Association and the National Heart, Lung and Blood Institute. *Circulation* 81, 1721-33, 1990.

10. Castelli WP and others. Cardiovascular risk factors in the elderly. *American Journal of Cardiology* 63, 12H-19H, 1989.

11. Claude Lenfant, Director of the National Heart, Lung and Blood Institute, answered a critical paper by the journalist Thomas Moore by claiming that, according to the Framingham study, high blood cholesterol was a risk factor for old people of both sexes. *The Atlantic Monthly*, January, p. 8, 1990.

12. Oliver MF. The optimum serum cholesterol. *The Lancet* 2, 655, 1982.

13. Forette B, Tortrat D, Wolmark Y. Cholesterol as risk factor for mortality in elderly women. *The Lancet* 1, 868-870, 1989. Ironically, in my practice it is usually old women who are most worried about their cholesterol level.

14. Jacobs D and others. Report of the conference on low blood cholesterol: *Circulation* 86, 1046-60, 1992.

15. Dagenais GR and others. Total and coronary heart disease mortality in relation to major risk factors - Quebec cardiovascular study. *Canadian Journal of Cardiology* 6, 59-65, 1990.

16. Shanoff HM, Little JA, Csima A. Studies of male survivors of myocardial infarction: XII. Relation of serum lipids and lipoproteins to survival over a 10-year period. *Canadian Medical Association Journal* 103, 927-931, 1970

17. a: Gertler MM and others. *American Journal of the Medical Sciences* 247, 145-155, 1964; b: Frank CW, Weinblatt E, Shapiro S. *Circulation* 47, 509-517, 1973; c: Mulcahy R and others. *British Heart Journal* 37, 158-165, 1975; d: Schatzkin A and others. *American Journal of Epidemiology* 120, 888-899, 1984; e: Khaw KT, Barrett-Connor E. *Journal of Cardiopulmonary Rehabilitation* 6, 474-480, 1986; f: Olsson G, Rehnqvist N. *Cardiology* 74, 457-464, 1987.

18. Carlson LA, Böttiger LE, Åhfeldt P-E. Risk factors for myocardial infarction in the Stockholm prospective study. *Acta Medica Scandinavica* 206, 351-360, 1979.

19. Böttiger LE, Carlson LA. Risk factors for death for males and females. *Acta Medica Scandinavica* 211, 437-442, 1982.

20. Beaglehole R and others. Cholesterol and mortality in New Zealand Maoris. *British Medical Journal* 1, 285-287, 1980.

21. Shestov DB and others. Increased risk of coronary heart disease death in men with low total and low-density-lipoprotein cholesterol in the Russian Lipid Research Clinics prevalence follow-up study. *Circulation* 88, 846-853, 1993.

22. Craig WE, Palomaki GE, Haddow JE. Cigarette smoking and serum lipid and lipoprotein concentrations: an analysis of published data. *British Medical Journal* 298, 784-788, 1989. This is a meta-analysis of 54 studies of lipid levels in smokers and non-smokers. Total cholesterol was 3 percent, VLDL 10.4 percent, LDL 1.7 percent and triglycerides 9.1 percent higher among smokers, and HDL 5.7 percent lower than among non-smokers. Interestingly, the authors thought that part of the explanation for the risk of smoking is its effects on the blood lipids; they did not consider the possibility that the changes of the blood levels may be secondary to the toxic effects of tobacco fumes. Their findings could as well mean that our bodies try to protect us against the fumes by producing more blood lipids. Thus, instead of being harmful, high cholesterol may be protective.

23. Dattilo AM, Kris-Etherton PM. Effects of weight reduction on blood lipids and lipoproteins: a meta-analysis. *American Journal of Clinical Nutrition* 56, 320-328, 1992.

24. Assmann G, Schulte H. The prospective cardiovascular Münster study: prevalence and prognostic significance of hyperlipidemia in men with systemic hypertension. *American Journal of Cardiology* 59, 9G-17G, 1987.

25. Dimsdale JE, Herd A. Variability of plasma lipids in response to emotional arousal. Psychosomatic Medicine 44, 413-430, 1982. Rosenman RH. Relationships of neurogenic and psychological factors to the regulation and variability of serum lipids. *Stress Medicine* 9, 133-140, 1993.

26. Even the Nobel Prize winners Joseph Goldstein and Michael Brown

have looked at Keys' illustrations only and mention only the great difference between Finland and Japan (Brown MS, Goldstein JL. How LDL-receptors influence cholesterol and atherosclerosis. *Scientific American* 251, 52-60, 1984).

27. Tuomilehto J, Kuulasmaa K. WHO MONICA Project: Assessing CHD mortality and morbidity. *International Journal of Epidemiology* 18, suppl. 1, S38-S45, 1989; Keil U, Kuulasmaa K. WHO MONICA Project: Risk factors. Same journal and issue: S46-S55.

28. On Corfu, the average cholesterol was 198 mg/dl, on Crete 202 mg/dl. Five-year incidence of coronary heart disease was 201 cases per 10,000 inhabitants on Corfu, 12 per 10,000 inhabitants on Crete. Note that these figures include all cases of coronary heart disease whereas Figure 2C includes only the number of fatal cases.

29. Keys A, and others. Lessons from serum cholesterol studies in Japan, Hawaii and Los Angeles. *Annals of Internal Medicine* 48, 83-94, 1958.

30. Worth RM and others. Epidemiologic studies of coronary heart disease and stroke in Japanese men living in Japan, Hawaii and California: mortality. *American Journal of Epidemiology* 102, 481-490, 1975.

31. (a) Marmot MG, Syme SL. Acculturation and coronary heart disease in Japanese-Americans. *American Journal of Epidemiology* 104, 225-247, 1976; (b) Marmot MG and others. Epidemiologic studies of coronary heart disease and stroke in Japanese men living in Japan, Hawaii and California: Prevalence of coronary and hypertensive heart disease and associated risk factors. *American Journal of Epidemiology* 102, 514-525, 1975.

32. Conference of the health effects of blood lipids: optimal distributions for populations. Workshop report: Epidemiological section. *Preventive Medicine* 8, 609-766, 1979.

33. Kannel WB, Doyle JT, Ostfeld AM, et al. Optimal resources for primary prevention of atherosclerotic diseases. *Circulation* 70, 157A-205A, 1984. The question is found on page 164A.

34. National Research Council. *Diet and Health. Implications for Reducing Chronic Disease Risk*. Washington D.C. 1989, National Academy Press. The quotation is found on page 166.

35. Ekelund LG and others. Physical fitness as a predictor of cardiovascular mortality in asymptomatic North American men. The Lipid Research Clinics' mortality follow-up study. *New England Journal of Medicine* 319, 1379-84, 1988.

36. Thompson PD and others. High-density lipoprotein metabolism in endurance athletes and sedentary men. *Circulation* 84, 140-152, 1991.

37. Pocock SJ and others. High-density lipoprotein cholesterol is not a major risk factor for ischaemic heart disease in British men. *British Medical Journal* 292, 515-519, 1986.

38. Gordon DJ and others. High-density lipoprotein cholesterol and cardiovascular disease. Four prospective American studies. *Circulation* 79, 8-15, 1989.

39. Pocock SJ, Shaper AG, Phillips AN. Concentrations of high-density lipoprotein cholesterol, triglycerides and total cholesterol in ischaemic

heart disease. *British Medical Journal* 298, 998-1002, 1989.

40. Keys A. and others. HDL serum cholesterol and 24-year mortality of men in Finland. *International Journal of Epidemiology* 13, 428-435, 1984.

41. Fumeron F and others. Lowering of HDL2-cholesterol and lipoprotein AI particle levels by increasing the ratio of polyunsaturated to saturated fatty acids. *American Journal of Clinical Nutrition* 53, 655-659, 1991.

42. Medalie JH and others. Five-year myocardial infarction incidence-II. Association of single variables to age and birthplace. *Journal of Chronic Diseases* 26, 329-349, 1973.

43. Gordon T and others. High density lipoprotein as a protective factor against coronary heart disease. *The American Journal of Medicine* 62, 707-714, 1977.

44. Watkins LO and others. Racial differences in high-density lipoprotein cholesterol and coronary heart disease incidence in the usual-care group of the multiple risk factor intervention trial. *American Journal of Cardiology* 57, 538-545, 1987.

45. The Expert Panel. Report of the National Cholesterol Education Program expert panel on detection, evaluation and treatment of high blood cholesterol in adults. *Archives of Internal Medicine* 148, 36-69, 1988.

46. Grundy SM. Cholesterol and coronary heart disease: a new era. *Journal of the American Medical Association* 256, 2849-2858, 1986.

47. Hulley SB, Rhoads GG. The plasma lipoproteins as risk factors: comparison of electrophoretic and ultracentrifugation results. *Metabolism* 31, 773-777, 1982.

48. Kannel WB and others. Optimal resources for primary prevention of atherosclerotic diseases. Atherosclerosis study group. *Circulation* 70, A157A-205A, 1984.

49. (a) Yaari and others. *The Lancet* 1, 1011-1015. 1981; (b) Keys A: *Seven Countries*. Harvard University Press, 1980.

50. (a) Rhoads GG, Gulbrandsen CL, Kagan A. Serum lipoproteins and coronary heart disease in a population study of Hawaii Japanese men. *New England Journal of Medicine* 294, 293-298, 1976; (b) The Pooling Project Research Group. Relationship of blood pressure, serum cholesterol, smoking habit, relative weight and ECG abnormalities to incidence of major coronary events: final report of the pooling project. *Journal of Chronic Diseases* 31, 201-306, 1978.

51. Conference on the health effects of blood lipids: optimal distributions for populations. *Preventive Medicine* 8, 612-678,1979, Tables 8-9.

52. Kannel WB, Castelli WP, Gordon T. Cholesterol in the prediction of atherosclerotic disease. New perspectives based on the Framingham study. *Annals of Internal Medicine* 90, 85-91, 1979.

53. Ravnskov U. Quotation bias in reviews of the diet-heart idea. *Journal of Clinical Epidemiology* 48, 713-719, 1995.

54. The Multiple Risk Factor Intervention Trial, the Newcastle Trial, the Lipid Research Clinics Trial, and the Helsinki Heart Study. For references to these studies, see Chapter 6, references 23, 25, 31, 38, 39.

55. Brown MS, Goldstein JL. How LDL receptors influence cholesterol and atherosclerosis. *Scientific American* 251, 58-66, 1984.

Chapter 3

1. Keys A and others. Lessons from serum cholesterol studies in Japan, Hawaii and Los Angeles. *Annals of Internal Medicine* 48, 83-94, 1958.
2. (a) Shaper AG. Cardiovascular studies in the Samburu tribe of northern Kenya. American Heart Journal 63, 437-442, 1962; (b) Shaper AG and others. Serum lipids in three nomadic tribes of northern Kenya. *American Journal of Clinical Nutrition* 13, 135-146, 1963.
3. Lapiccirella V and others. Enquête clinique, biologique et cardiographique parmi les tribus nomades de la Somalie qui se nourissent seulement de lait. *Bulletin of the World Health Organization* 27, 681-697, 1962.
4. Prior IA and others. Cholesterol, coconuts and diet on Polynesian atolls: a natural experiment: the Pukapuka and Tokelau Island studies. *American Journal of Clinical Nutrition* 34, 1552-1561, 1981.
5. Stanhope JM, Sampson VM, Prior IAM. The Tokelau Island migrant study: serum lipid concentrations in two environments. *Journal of Chronic Disease* 34, 45-55, 1980.
6. Ramsay LE, Yeo WW, Jackson PR. Dietary reduction of serum cholesterol concentration: time to think again. *British Medical Journal* 303, 953-957, 1991.
7. According to a personal communication from George Mann, who was the director of this part of the Framingham study. George Mann left the project after three years before all data had been gathered.
8. Nichols AB and others. Daily nutritional intake and serum lipid levels. The Tecumseh study. *American Journal of Clinical Nutrition* 29, 1384-1392, 1976.
9. Weidman WH and others. Nutrient intake and serum cholesterol level in normal children 6 to 16 years of age. *Pediatrics* 61, 354-359, 1978.
10. Frank GC, Berenson GS, Webber LS. Dietary studies and the relationship of diet to cardiovascular disease risk factor variables in 10-year-old children—the Bogalusa heart study. *The American Journal of Clinical Nutrition* 31, 328-340, 1978. After dividing the children into three groups according to their blood cholesterol values, the researchers found that the children with the lowest values ate less fat, both saturated and unsaturated, than the children with the intermediate and the highest cholesterol values. No difference was found between the two latter groups. The ratio between saturated and polyunsaturated fat was almost identical in all groups, however. This ratio, considered the best measure of the effect of dietary fat on blood cholesterol, was not calculated in the tables, nor was it mentioned in the text. Here the authors admitted on the one hand that the diet possibly played only a minor role in the development of atherosclerosis; on the other hand they said there was, "as might be expected," a relationship between saturated fat and blood cholesterol. And they added that "such studies do reinforce

the need for seriously considering general modifications of food patterns at a young age."

11. Morris JN and others. Diet and plasma cholesterol in 99 bank men.
British Medical Journal 1, 571-576, 1963.

12. Kroneld R, and others. Hälsobeteende och riskfaktorer för hjärt-och
kärlsjukdomar i östra och sydvästra Finland. *Suomen Lääkarilehti*
45, 735-739, 1990.

13. Kahn HA and others. Serum cholesterol: Its distribution and association with dietary and other variables in a survey of 10,000 men. *Israel
Journal of the Medical Sciences* 5, 1117-1127, 1969. Stamler's group
performed a similar study on 1900 middle-aged men. This study is
impossible for anyone but statisticians to evaluate, since absolute figures were absent, and not even simple correlation coefficients were
given. The relationship between the diet and the risk of dying from
CHD after the age of 19 was also studied, but again without giving any
figures. The amount of saturated fat in the diet did not show any relationship with the risk of dying from CHD, the authors admitted, but
they added that it was not possible to draw conclusions from only one
study; if their results were seen "within the context of the total literature," they supported the diet-heart idea. (Shekelle RB and others.
Diet, serum cholesterol, and death from coronary heart disease. The
Western Electric Study. *New England Journal of Medicine* 304, 65-70,
1981).

14. Balogh M, Kahn HA, Medalie JH. Random repeat 24-hour dietary re-
calls. *American Journal of Clinical Nutrition* 24, 304-310, 1971.

15. Hopkins PN. Effects of dietary cholesterol on serum cholesterol: a
meta-analysis and review. *American Journal of Clinical Nutrition* 55,
1060-1070, 1992.

16. Katan MB and others. Existence of consistent hypo- and hyper-
responders to dietary cholesterol in man. *American Journal of Epidemiology* 123, 221-234, 1986.

Chapter 4

1.   Keys A. Atherosclerosis, a problem in newer public health. *Journal of
the Mount Sinai Hospital* New York 20, 118-139, 1953.

2.   Landé KE, Sperry WM. Human atherosclerosis in relation to the cholesterol content of the blood serum. *Archives of Pathology* 22, 301-
312, 1936.

3.   Epstein FH, Ostrander LD. Detection of individual susceptibility toward coronary disease. *Progress of Cardiovascular Diseases* 13, 324-
342, 1971: "An association between cholesterol concentration and coronary atherosclerosis was also recognized among individuals without
the extreme manifestations of typical hyperlipidemia or hyper-cholesterolemia," the authors wrote, a statement in conflict with Landé's and
Sperry's data and conclusions.

4.   Paterson JC, Armstrong R, Armstrong EC. Serum lipid levels and the

severity of coronary and cerebral atherosclerosis in adequately nourished men, 60 to 69 years of age. *Circulation* 27, 229-236, 1963.

5. Mathur KS and others. Serum cholesterol and atherosclerosis in man. *Circulation* 23, 847-852, 1961.

6. Marek Z, Jaegermann K, Ciba T. Atherosclerosis and levels of serum cholesterol in postmortem investigations. *American Heart Journal* 63, 768-774, 1962.

7. Méndez J, Tejada C. Relationship between serum lipids and aortic atherosclerotic lesions in sudden accidental deaths in Guatemala City. *American Journal of Clinical Nutrition* 20, 1113-1117, 1967.

8. Cabin HS, Roberts WC. Relation of serum total cholesterol and triglyceride levels to the amount and extent of coronary arterial narrowing by atherosclerotic plaque in coronary heart disease. *American Journal of Medicine* 73, 227-234, 1982.

9. Feinleib M and others. The relation of antemortem characteristics to cardiovascular findings at necropsy. *The Framingham Study. Atherosclerosis.* 34, 145-157, 1979.

10. Okumiya N and others. Coronary and antecedent risk factors: Pathologic and epidemiologic study in Hisayama, Japan. *American Journal of Cardiology* 56, 62-66, 1985.

11. Hatano S, Matsuzaki T. Atherosclerosis in relation to personal attributes of a Japanese population in homes for the aged. *International Symposium of Atherosclerosis IV*. Edit.: Schettler G, Goto Y, Hata Y, Klose G. Springer-Verlag, New York, 1977, p. 116-120.

12. Solberg LA and others. Stenoses in the coronary arteries. The Oslo study. *Laboratory Investigation* 53, 648-655, 1985. Unsystematic relationships, selected autopsy studies and low correlation coefficients were also found in the following papers: Rhoads GG and others. Coronary risk factors and autopsy findings in Japanese-American men. *Laboratory Investigation* 38, 304-311, 1978 and Reed DM and others. Serum lipids and lipoproteins as predictors of atherosclerosis. An autopsy study. *Atherosclerosis* 9, 560-564, 1989.

13. Pearson TA. Coronary arteriography in the study of the epidemiology of coronary artery disease. *Epidemiological Reviews.* 6, 140-166, 1984. In his review Pearson mentions a number of angiographic studies that he claimed had found a relationship between blood cholesterol levels and degrees of atherosclerosis. But three of them found no relationship; one of these is reference number 14 (see the text), the other two are: Nitter-Hauge S, Enge I. Relation between blood lipid levels and angiographically evaluated obstructions in coronary arteries. *British Heart Journal* 35, 791-795, 1973 and Barboriak JJ and others. Coronary artery occlusion and blood lipids. *American Heart Journal* 87, 716-721, 1974. An unsupportive study was ignored by Pearson: Fuster V and others. Arteriographic patterns early in the onset of the coronary syndromes. *British Heart Journal* 37, 1250-1255, 1975.

14. Cramér K, Paulin S, Werkö L. Coronary angiographic findings in correlation with age, body weight, blood pressure, serum lipids and smoking habits. *Circulation* 33, 888-900, 1966.

15. Bemis CE, and others. Progression of coronary artery disease. A clinical arteriographic study. *Circulation* 47, 455-464, 1973.
16. Kimbiris D and others. Devolutionary pattern of coronary atherosclerosis in patients with angina pectoris. Coronary arteriographic studies. *American Journal of Cardiology* 33, 7-11, 1974.
17. Shub C and others. The unpredictable progression of symptomatic coronary artery disease. *Mayo Clinic Proceedings* 56, 155-160, 1981.
18. (a) McLaughlin PR and others. Long-term angiographic assessment of the influence of coronary risk factors on native coronary circulation and saphenous vein aortocoronary grafts. *American Heart Journal* 93, 327-333, 1977; (b) Merchandise B and others. Angiographic evaluation of the natural history of normal coronary arteries and mild coronary atherosclerosis. *American Journal of Cardiology* 41, 216-220, 1978; (c) Kramer JR and others. Progression and regression of coronary atherosclerosis: relation to risk factors. *American Heart Journal* 105, 134-144, 1983.
19. Waters D, Craven TE, Lespérance J. Prognostic significance of progression of coronary atherosclerosis. *Circulation* 87, 1067-1075, 1993.
20. (a) Cohn K and others. Effect of clofibrate on progression of coronary disease: a prospective angiographic study in man. *American Heart Journal.* 89, 591-598, 1975; (b) Arntzenius AC and others. Diet, lipoproteins, and the progression of coronary atherosclerosis. The Leiden Intervention Trial. *New England Journal of Medicine* 312, 805-811, 1985; (c) Krauss RM and others. Intermediate-density lipoproteins and progression of coronary artery disease in hypercholesterolaemic men. *The Lancet* 2, 62-66, 1987; (d) Blankenhorn DH and others. Prediction of angiographic change in native human coronary arteries and aortocoronary bypass grafts. Lipid and nonlipid factors. *Circulation* 81, 470-476, 1990; (e) Brown G and others. Regression of coronary artery disease as a result of intensive lipid-lowering therapy in men with high levels of apolipoprotein B. *New England Journal of Medicine* 323, 1289-1298, 1990; (f) Tatami R and others. Regression of coronary atherosclerosis by combined LDL-apheresis and lipid-lowering drug therapy in patients with familial hypercholesterolemia: a multicenter study. *Atherosclerosis* 95, 1-13, 1992; (g) Hambrecht R and others. Various intensities of leisure time physical activity in patients with coronary artery disease: effects on cardiorespiratory fitness and progression of coronary atherosclerotic lesions. *Journal of the American College of Cardiology* 22, 468-477, 1993; (h) Hodis HN and others. Triglyceride- and cholesterol-rich lipoproteins have a differential effect on mild/moderate and severe lesion progression as assessed by quantitative coronary angiography in a controlled trial of lovastatin. *Circulation* 90:42-49, 1994; (i) Sacks FM and others. Effect on coronary atherosclerosis of decrease in plasma cholesterol concentrations in normocholesterolaemic patients. *The Lancet* 344, 1182-1186, 1994; (j) Quinn TG and others. Development of new coronary atherosclerotic lesions during a 4-year multifactor risk reduction program: The Stanford coronary risk reduction project (SCRIP). *Journal of the Ameri-*

can College of Cardiology 24, 900-908, 1994; (k) Schuff-Werner P and others. The HELP-LDL-apheresis multicentre study, an angiographically assessed trial on the role of LDL-apheresis in the secondary prevention of coronary heart disease. II. Final evaluation of the effect of regular treatment on LDL-cholesterol plasma concentrations and the course of coronary heart disease. *European Journal of Clinical Investigation* 24, 724-732, 1994; (l) Kitabatake A and others. Coronary atherosclerosis reduced in patients with familial hypercholesterolemia after intensive cholesterol lowering with low-density lipoprotein-apheresis: 1-year follow-up study. *Clinical Therapy* 16, 416-428, 1994; (m) Niebauer J and others. Predictive value of lipid profile for salutary coronary angiographic changes in patients on a low-fat diet and physical exercise program. *American Journal of Cardiology* 78, 163-167, 1996; (n) Kroop AA and others. LDL-apheresis atherosclerosis regression study (LAARS). Effect of aggressive versus conventional lipid lowering treatment on coronary atherosclerosis. *Circulation* 93, 1826-1835, 1996; (o) Tamura A and others. Effect of Pravastatin (10 mg/day) on progression of coronary atherosclerosis in patients with serum total cholesterol levels from 160 to 220 mg/dl and angiographically documented coronary disease. *American Journal of Cardiology* 79, 893-896, 1997; (p) Ruotolo G and others. Treatment effects on serum lipoprotein lipids, apolipoproteins and low density lipoprotein particle size and relationships of lipoprotein variables to progression of coronary artery disease in the bezafibrate coronary atherosclerosis intervention trial (BECAIT). *Journal of the American College of Cardiology* 32, 1648-1656, 1998; (q) Sutherland WHF and others. IDL composition and angiographically determined progression of atherosclerotic lesions during simvastatin therapy. *Arteriosclerosis* 18, 577-583, 1998; (r) Bemis CE and others. Progression of coronary artery disease. A clinical arteriographic study. *Circulation* 47:455-464, 1973; (s) Shub C and others. The unpredictable progression of symptomatic coronary artery disease. A serial clinical-angiographic analysis. *Mayo Clinic Proceedings* 56:155-160, 1981; (t) Kramer JR and others. Progression and regression of coronary atherosclerosis: relation to risk factors. *American Heart Journal* 105:134-144, 1983; (u) Bruschke AVG and others. The dynamics of progression of coronary atherosclerosis studied in 168 medically treated patients who underwent coronary arteriography three times. *American Heart Journal* 117, 296-305, 1989; (v) Bissett JK and others. Plasma lipid concentrations and subsequent coronary occlusion after a first myocardial infarction. *American Journal of the Clinical Sciences* 305, 139-144, 1993.

21. Gore I, Hirst AE, Koseki Y. Comparison of aortic atherosclerosis in the United States, Japan, and Guatemala. *American Journal of Clinical Nutrition* 7, 50-54, 1959.

22. Resch JA, Okabe N, Kimoto K. Cerebral atherosclerosis. *Geriatrics* November, p. 111-132, 1969.

Chapter 5

1. (a) Lindsay S, Chaikoff IL. Naturally occurring arteriosclerosis in animals: a comparison with experimentally induced lesions. In Sandler M, Bourne GH. (ed) Atherosclerosis and its origin. Academic Press, New York 1963, p 349-437; (b) Detweiler DK, Ratcliffe HL, Luginbühl H. The significance of naturally occurring coronary and cerebral arterial disease in animals. *Annals of the New York Academy of Science* 149, 868-881, 1968.
2. (a) Vastesaeger MM. The contribution of comparative atherosclerosis to the understanding of human atherosclerosis. *Journal of Atherosclerosis Research* 8, 377-380, 1968; (b) Stout C, Groover ME. Spontaneous versus experimental atherosclerosis. *Annals of the New York Academy of Science* 162, 89-98, 1969; (c) Stout LC, Bohorquez MS. Significance of intimal arterial changes in non-human vertebrates. *Medical Clinics of North America* 58, 245-255, 1974; (d) Stehbens WE. An appraisal of cholesterol feedings in experimental atherogenesis. *Progress of Cardiovascular Research* 29, 107-128, 1986; (e) Stehbens WE. Vascular complications in experimental atherosclerosis. *Progress of Cardiovascular Research* 29, 221-237, 1986.
3. Taylor CB, Manalo-Estrella P, Southworth J. Atherosclerosis in rhesus monkeys. II. Arterial lesions associated with hypercholesterolemia induced by dietary fat and cholesterol. *Archives of Pathology* 74, 16-34, 1962.
4. Taylor CB, Patton DE, Cox GE. Atherosclerosis in rhesus monkeys. VI. Fatal myocardial infarction in a monkey fed fat and cholesterol. *Archives of Pathology* 76, 404-412, 1963.
5. Kramsch DM and others. Reduction of coronary atherosclerosis by moderate conditioning exercise in monkeys on an atherogenic diet. *New England Journal of Medicine* 305, 1483-1489, 1981.

Chapter 6

1. Cornfield J, Mitchell S. Selected risk factors in coronary disease. *Archives of Environmental Health* 19, 382-394, 1969.
2. Report of a research committee to the medical research council. Controlled trial of soya-bean oil in myocardial infarction. *The Lancet* 2, 693-700, 1968.
3. Leren P. The effect of plasma cholesterol-lowering diet in male survivors of myocardial infarction. *Acta Medica Scandinavica* Suppl. 466, 1966.
4. Dayton S and others. A controlled clinical trial of a diet high in unsaturated fat in preventing complications of atherosclerosis. *Circulation* 40, suppl. II, 1-63, 1969. The mean reduction of blood cholesterol was 12.7 percent. In the control group 70 died from atherosclerotic vascular disease against 48 in the soybean oil group. But more died from other causes, especially from cancer; thus the total number of deaths was almost equal, 174 against 177, and there were more heavy smok-

ers in the control group.

5.   The Coronary Drug Project Research Group. The coronary drug project. Design, methods and baseline results. *Circulation* 47, suppl. 1, 1-50, 1973.

6.   *Ibid.* Initial findings leading to modifications of its research protocol. *Journal of the American Medical Association* 214, 1303-1313, 1970.

7.   *Ibid.* Findings leading to discontinuation of the 2.5-mg/day estrogen group. *Journal of the American Medical Association* 226, 652-657, 1973.

8.   *Ibid.* Findings leading to further modifications of its protocol with respect to dextrothyroxine. *Journal of the American Medical Association* 220, 996-1008, 1972.

9.   Ibid. Clofibrate and niacin in coronary heart disease. *Journal of the American Medical Association* 231, 360-381, 1975.

10. 10.2 percent non-lethal heart attacks in the nicotinic acid group against 13.8 percent in the control group. Information about the number of suspect heart attacks was absent. This is not unimportant because the diagnosis "heart attack" is often doubtful; a more critical approach may have been used unintentionally in the nicotinic acid group. Information about both certain and suspect cases of cerebral thrombosis and stroke was given, however.

11. Canner PL and others. Fifteen-year mortality in coronary drug project patients: long-term benefit with niacin. *Journal of the American College of Cardiology* 8, 1245-1255, 1986.

12. Dorr AE and others. Colestipol hydrochloride in hypercholesterolemic patients—effect on serum cholesterol and mortality. *Journal of Chronic Disease* 31, 5-14, 1978.

13. Blood triglycerides in the placebo group were 220 mg%, in the treatment group 284 mg%. A difference of this magnitude demonstrates that the randomization of the test individuals has failed. As the directors of the trial had access to the blood triglyceride values of the participants, they might, intentionally or not, have placed more individuals with familial hypercholesterolemia (blood triglyceride is normal in this condition) in the control group. The best method of separating patients and controls in a trial is called random allocation. This implies that the test individuals are divided randomly, for instance, by day of birth, or by following a computerized allocation program. If the number of test individuals is as large as in the Upjohn trial, chance will distribute any risk factor haphazardly and thus minimize the risk of bias.

14. The primary results from the WHO trial are found in *British Heart Journal* 40, 1069-1118, 1978, the follow-up results in *The Lancet* 2, 379-385, 1980.

15. Salonen JT, Puska P, Mustaniemi H. Changes in morbidity and mortality during comprehensive community programme to control cardiovascular disease during 1972-7 in North Karelia. *British Medical Journal* 2, 1178-1183, 1979.

16. (a) Salonen JT. Primary prevention of sudden coronary death: a com-

munity-based program in North Karelia, Finland. *Annals of the New York Academy of Science* 382, 423-437, 1982; (b) Tuomilehto J and others. Decline in cardiovascular mortality in North Karelia and other parts of Finland. *British Medical Journal* 293, 1068-1071, 1986.
17. Salonen JT. Did the North Karelia project reduce coronary mortality? *The Lancet* 2, 269, 1987.
18. Oliver MF. North Karelia project. *The Lancet* 2, 518, 1987.
19. *Hufvudstadsbladet* 23. juni 1988.
20. Hjermann I, Byre KV, Holme I, Leren P. Effect of diet and smoking intervention on the incidence of coronary heart disease. Report from the Oslo study group of a randomized trial in healthy men. *The Lancet* 2, 1303-10, 1981.
21. The weight loss in the treatment group is easily overlooked because body weight was not given in kilograms but in relative body weight (body weight divided by the square of body height):

| | Relative Body Weight | |
	Before	After
Treatment group	24.44	23.28
Control group	25.46	25.65

The figures are equivalent to an approximate weight difference of 6-7 kilograms after the treatment period.
22. Kannel WB. New perspectives on cardiovascular risk factors. *American Heart Journal* 114, 213-219, 1987.
23. Increased mortality after lipid-lowering diets was seen in the following experiments: (a) Rose GA and others. Corn oil in the treatment of ischemic heart disease. *British Medical Journal* 1, 1531-1533, 1965; (b) Woodhill JM and others. Low-fat, low-cholesterol diet in secondary prevention of coronary heart disease. *Advances of Experimental and Medical Biology* 109, 317-330, 1978. No difference was found in these experiments: a: Research Committee to the Medical Research Council: Low-fat diet in myocardial infarction: A controlled trial. *The Lancet* 2, 501-504, 1965; (c) Research Committee to the Medical Research Council: Controlled trial of soya-bean oil in myocardial infarction. *The Lancet* 2, 693-700, 1968; (d) Research Committee of the Scottish Society of Physicians: Ischaemic Heart Disease: a secondary prevention trial using clofibrate. *British Medical Journal* 4, 775-784, 1971. The only experiment in which mortality was lowered was: de Lorgeril M and others. Mediterranean diet, traditional risk factors, and the rate of cardiovascular complications after myocardial infarction. Final report of the Lyon Diet Heart Study. *Circulation* 99, 779-785, 1993.
24. The coronary primary prevention trial: design and implementation. *Journal of Chronic Disease* 32, 609-631, 1979.
25. The results from the first seven years of MRFIT were published in *Journal of the American Medical Association* 248, 1465-1477, 1982 and in *American Journal of Cardiology* 58, 1-13, 1986.

26. The pilot study was published in *Circulation* 37, suppl. I, 1-428, 1968; figures of the diet and blood cholesterol in the multiple risk factor intervention trial (MRFIT). IV. Intervention on blood lipids. *Preventive Medicine* 10, 443-475, 1981; table IX,1 and table XII,e.
27. *Journal of the American Medical Association* 248, 1465-1477, 1982.
28. In fact, the smoking habits explained the whole difference. This is best demonstrated by simplifying a complicated table in the *JAMA* paper in the following way (table 9) :

	Treatment Group		Control Group	
	Number	Coronary Mortality	Number	Coronary Mortality
Ceased smoking	991	11.1%	374	10.7%
Continued	2842	20.4%	3456	20.3%

If the table is read horizontally, the effect of the diet is seen. If it is read vertically, the effect of quitting smoking is seen. Thus, the table shows that it does not matter what you eat, but coronary mortality is cut in half if you stop smoking.
29. Mortality rates after 10.5 years for participants in the multiple risk factor intervention trial. *Journal of the American Medical Association* 263, 1795-1801, 1990.
30. *Journal of the American Dietetic Association* 86, 744-758, 1986.
31. The Lipid Research Clinic's coronary primary prevention trial results. 1. Reduction in incidence of coronary heart disease. *Journal of the American Medical Association* 251, 351-64, 1984.
32. The coronary primary prevention trial: design and implementation. *Journal of Chronic Disease* 32, 609-631, 1979. Criticism of the change of the statistical demands was published in the *Journal of the American Medical Association* 253, 3091, 1985, together with the response from the trial directors.
33. A two-tailed t-test is much more difficult to satisfy than a one-tailed test, and it is therefore more reliable. Scientists have agreed that a one-tailed t-test should be used only when it is certain that the result will go in just one direction. The one-tailed t-test is never to be used when a study—for instance, a drug trial, where the drug may do harm rather than good—may have a negative as well as a positive outcome.
34. *Journal of the American Medical Association* 253, 3091, 1985.
35. *The Atlantic Monthly*, January 1990.
36. *British Medical Journal* 301, 815, 1990.
37. Miettinen TA and others. Multifactorial primary prevention of cardiovascular diseases in middle-aged men. *Journal of the American Medical Association* 254, 2097-2102, 1985.
38. Frick MH and 18 others. Helsinki heart study: Primary-prevention trial with gemfibrozil in middle-aged men with dyslipidemia. *New England Journal of Medicine* 317, 1237-1245, 1987.

39. Frick MH and others. Efficacy of gemfibrozil in dyslipaemic subjects with suspected heart disease. An ancillary study in the Helsinki heart study frame population. *Annals of Medicine* 25, 41-45, 1993.

40. Koivisto P, Miettinen TA. Long-term effects of ileal bypass on lipoproteins in patients with familial hypercholesterolemia. *Circulation* 70, 290-296, 1984.

41. Buchwald H and others. Effect of partial ileal bypass surgery on mortality and morbidity from coronary heart disease in patients with hypercholesterolemia. Report of the program on the surgical control of the hyperlipidemias (POSCH). *New England Journal of Medicine* 323, 946-955, 1990.

42. Brensike JF and 14 others. Effects of therapy with cholestyramine on progression of coronary atherosclerosis: results of the NHLBI type II coronary intervention study. *Circulation* 69, 313-324, 1984.

43. Levy RI and 14 others. The influence of changes in lipid values induced by cholestyramine and diet on progression of coronary artery disease: results of the NHLBI type II coronary intervention study. *Circulation* 69, 325-337, 1984.

44. Blankenhorn DH and others. Beneficial effects of combined colestipol-niacin therapy on coronary atherosclerosis and coronary venous bypass grafts. *Journal of the American Medical Association* 257, 3233-3240, 1987.

45. Roberts L. Study bolsters case against cholesterol. *Science* 237, 28-29, 1987. An ironic description of the marketing of the CLAS trial.

46. Brown G and others. Regression of coronary artery disease as a result of intensive lipid-lowering therapy in men with high levels of apolipoprotein B. *New England Journal of Medicine* 323, 1289-98, 1990.

47. Brown G and others. Reflex constriction of significant coronary stenosis as a mechanism contributing to ischemic left ventricular dysfunction during isometric exercise. *Circulation* 70, 18-24, 1984.

48. Glagov S and others. Compensatory enlargement of human atherosclerotic coronary arteries. *New England Journal of Medicine* 316, 1371-1375, 1987.

49. Ravnskov U. Cholesterol-lowering trials in coronary heart disease: frequency of citation and outcome. *British Medical Journal* 305, 15-19, 1992

50. *British Medical Journal* 305, 420-422, 1992.

51. Stamler J and others. Effectiveness of estrogens for therapy of myocardial infarction in middle age men. *Journal of the American Medical Association* 183, 632-638, 1963.

52. Stampfer MJ and others. Postmenopausal estrogen therapy and cardiovascular disease. Ten-year follow-up from the nurses' health study. *New England Journal of Medicine* 325, 756-62, 1991.

53. Davey Smith G, Song F, Sheldon TA. Cholesterol lowering and mortality: the importanc of considering initial level of risk. *British Medical Journal* 306, 1367-1373, 1993.

54. International Task Force for Prevention of Coronary Heart Disease.

Prevention of coronary heart disease: Scientific background and new clinical guidelines. *Nutrition, Metabolism and Cardiovascular Diseases* 2, 113-156, 1992. Recall that the citation is from a paper written before the statin trials were published.

55. de Lorgeril M and others. Mediterranean alpha-linolenic acid-rich diet in secondary prevention of coronary heart disease. *The Lancet* 343, 1454-1459, 1994.

56. Sandker GW and others. Serum cholesterol ester fatty acids and their relation with serum lipids in elderly men in Crete and the Netherlands. *European Journal of Clinical Nutrition* 47, 201-208, 1993.

57. de Lorgeril M and others. Mediterranean diet, traditional risk factors, and the rate of cardiovascular complications after myocardial infarction. Final report of the Lyon Diet Heart Study. *Circulation* 99, 779-785, 1993

58. Ascherio A and others. Dietary fat and risk of coronary heart disease in men: cohort follow-up study in the United States. *British Medical Journal* 313, 84-90, 1996.

59. Leng GC and others. Essential fatty acids and cardiovascular disease: the Edinburgh Artery Study. *Vascular Medicine* 4, 219-226, 1999.

60. Guallar E and others. Omega-3 fatty acids in adipose tissue and risk of myocardial infarction: the EURAMIC study. *Arteriosclerosis, Thrombosis and Vascular Biology* 19, 1111-1118, 1999.

61. Scandinavian Simvastatin Survival Study Group. Randomised trial of cholesterol lowering in 4444 patients with coronary heart disease: the Scandinavian Simvastatin Survival Study (4S). *The Lancet* 344, 1383-1389, 1994.

62. Oliver M, Poole-Wilson P, Shepherd J, Tikkanen MJ. Lower patients' cholesterol now. Trial evidence shows clear benefits from secondary prevention. *British Medical Journal* 310, 1280-1281, 1995.

63. Sacks FM and others. The effect of pravastatin on coronary events after myocardial infarction in patients with average cholesterol levels. *New England Journal of Medicine* 335, 1001-1009, 1996.

64. Shepherd J. and others Prevention of coronary disease with pravastatin in men with hypercholesterolemia. *New England Journal of Medicine* 333, 1301-1307, 1995.

65. Downs JR and others. Primary prevention of acute coronary events with lovastatin in men and women with average cholesterol levels. Results of AFCAPS/TexCAPS. *Journal of the American Medical Association* 279, 1615-1622, 1998.

66. The Long-Term Intervention with Pravastatin in Ischaemic Disease (LIPID) Study Group. Prevention of cardiovascular events and death with pravastatin in patients with coronary heart disease and a broad range of initial cholesterol levels. *New England Journal of Medicine* 339, 1349-1357, 1998.

67. The following studies did not find that a high cholesterol is a risk factor for a new heart attack: Gertler MM et al. *American Journal of Medical Science* 247, 145-155, 1964. Shanoff HM, Little JA, Csima A. *Canadian Medical Association Journal* 103, 927-931, 1970. Frank CW,

Weinblatt E, Shapiro S. *Circulation* 47, 509-517, 1973. Mulcahy R et al. *British Heart Journal* 37, 158-165, 1975. Schatzkin A et al. *American Journal of Epidemiology* 129, 888-899, 1984. Khaw KT, Barrett-Connor E. *Journal of Cardiopulmonary Rehabilitation* 6, 474-480, 1986. Olsson G, Rehnqvist N. *Cardiology* 74, 457-64, 1987.

There are ten studies where the relationship was weak, dichotomized or unsystematic; only in three studies a strong and graded, positive correlation was found: Rose et al. *The Lancet* 1, 105-109, 1977. Pekkanen J et al. *New England Journal of Medicine* 322, 1700-1707, 1990. Phillips AN et al. *British Heart Journal* 60, 404-410, 1988.

68. When the results from the first statin trial, the 4S Study, were presented for Swedish doctors, one of the striking findings was the lack of exposure-response, both for total and LDL-cholesterol. I was present at two of the meetings and pointed out this striking deviation from the cholesterol hypothesis. On both occasions, it was obvious that the speakers had not recognized the implications of this phenomenon. It was not mentioned either in the first report published in *The Lancet* in 1994. Four years later a new report was published that demonstrated exposure-response. (Pedersen T and others. Lipoprotein changes and reduction in the incidence of major coronary heart disease events in the Scandinavian Simvastatin Survival Study (4S). *Circulation* 97, 1453-1460, 1998.) However, this report concerned only the first year of the trial. In a letter published in a Swedish medical journal (*Läkartidningen* 96, 1948-1949, 1999), I asked one of the authors, Professor Anders G. Olsson, to explain why they had published the exposure-response calculations for the first year but not for the whole trial. He did not answer.

69. Ravnskov U. Implications of 4S evidence on baseline lipid levels. *The Lancet* 346, 102-103, 1995. Massy ZA, Keane WF, Kasiske BL. Inhibition of the mevalonate pathway: benefits beyond cholesterol reduction? *The Lancet* 347, 102-103, 1996. Vaughan CJ, Murphy MB, Buckley BM. Statins do more than just lower cholesterol? *The Lancet* 348, 1079-1082, 1996.

70. Soma MR, Corsini A, Paoletti R. Cholesterol and mevalonic acid modulation in cell metabolism and multiplication. *Toxicology Letters* 64/65, 1-15, 1992.

71. Hidaka Y, Eda T, Yonemoto M, Kamei T. Inhibition of cultured vascular smooth muscle cell migration by simvastatin (MK-733). *Atherosclerosis* 95, 87-94, 1992.

72. (a) Tremoli E, Folco G, Agradi E, Galli C. Platelet thromboxanes and serum-cholesterol. *The Lancet* 1, 107-8, 1979; (b) Schrör K. Platelet reactivity and arachidonic acid metabolism in type II hyperlipoproteinaemia and its modification by cholesterol-lowering agents. *Eicosanoids* 3, 67-73, 1990; (c) Davi G, and others. Increased thromboxane biosynthesis in type IIa hypercholesterolemia. *Circulation* 85, 1792-8, 1992.

73. Meiser BM and others. Simvastatin decreases accelerated graft vessel disease after heart transplantation in an animal model. *Transplanta-*

tion Proceedings 25, 2077-9, 1993.
74. Soma MR and others. HMG CoA reductase inhibitors. In vivo effects on carotid intimal thickening in normocholesterolemic rabbits. *Atherosclerosis* 13, 571-8, 1993.
75. Newman TB, Hulley SB. Carcinogenicity of lipid-lowering drugs. *Journal of the American Medical Association* 27, 55-60, 1996.
76. Bradford RH and others. Expanded clinical evaluation of lovastatin (EXCEL) study results. *Archives of Internal Medicine* 151, 43-49, 1991.
77. I asked that question to Merck, Sharp & Dohme. They answered that the trial was not designed to measure the clinical outcome, only to test whether the drug was tolerable and did not produce any serious side effects.
78. Executive Summary of the third report of the National Cholesterol Education Program (NCEP)expert panel on detection,evaluation, and treatment of high blood cholesterol in adults (adult treatment panel III). *Journal of the American Medical Association* 285, 2486-97, 2001.
79. Hecht HS,Superko HR.Electron beam tomography and National Cholesterol Education Program guidelines in asymptomatic women. *Journal of the American College of Cardiology* 37, 1506-1511, 2001.
80. Most of the authors of the guidelines are, like almost all cholesterol researchers, supported financially by the drug companies. Here follows a list, given by themselves to the *Journal of the American Medical Association*[1]: Financial Disclosure: Dr Grundy has received honoraria from Merck, Pfizer, Sankyo, Bayer, and Bristol-Myers Squibb. Dr Hunninghake has current grants from Merck, Pfizer, Kos Pharmaceuticals, Schering Plough, Wyeth Ayerst, Sankyo, Bayer, AstraZeneca, Bristol-Myers Squibb, and G. D. Searle; he has also received consulting honoraria from Merck, Pfizer, Kos Pharmaceuticals, Sankyo, AstraZeneca, and Bayer. Dr McBride has received grants and/or research support from Pfizer, Merck, Parke-Davis, and AstraZeneca; has served as a consultant for Kos Pharmaceuticals, Abbott, and Merck; and has received honoraria from Abbott, Bristol-Myers Squibb, Novartis, Merck, Kos Pharmaceuticals, Parke-Davis, Pfizer, and DuPont. Dr Pasternak has served as a consultant for and received honoraria from Merck, Pfizer, and Kos Pharmaceuticals, and has received grants from Merck and Pfizer. Dr Stone has served as a consultant and/or received honoraria for lectures from Abbott, Bayer, Bristol-Myers Squibb, Kos Pharmaceuticals, Merck, Novartis, Parke-Davis/Pfizer, and Sankyo. Dr Schwartz has served as a consultant for and/or conducted research funded by Bristol-Myers Squibb, AstraZeneca, Merck, Johnson & Johnson-Merck, and Pfizer.
81. A review of five prospective studies of vegetarians and nonvegetarians found that a significantly lower mortality in coronary heart disease was balanced by a higher mortality in other diseases, resulting in a total mortality among the vegetarians that did not differ from the total mortality of nonvegetarians. Key TJ and others. Mortality in vegetarians and nonvegetarians: detailed findings from a collaborative analysis of 5 prospective studies. *American Journal of Clinical Nutrition*, 70(suppl). 516S-524S, 1999.

Chapter 7

1. (a) Stemmermann GN and others. Serum cholesterol and colon cancer
    incidence in Hawaiian-Japanese men. *Journal of the National Cancer
    Institute* 67, 1179-1182, 1981; (b) Morris DL and others. Serum cho-
    lesterol and cancer in the hypertension detection and follow-up pro-
    gram. *Cancer* 52, 1754-1759, 1983; (c) Sherwin RW and others. Se-
    rum cholesterol levels and cancer mortality in 361,662 men screened
    for the multiple risk factor intervention trial. *Journal of the American
    Medical Association* 257, 943-948, 1987; (d) Isles CG and others. Plasma
    cholesterol, coronary heart disease, and cancer in the Renfrew and
    Paisley survey. *British Medical Journal* 298, 920-924, 1989; (e) Winawer
    SJ, and others. Declining serum cholesterol levels prior to diagnosis
    of colon cancer. A time-trend, case-control study. *Journal of the Ameri-
    can Medical Association* 263, 2083-2085, 1990; (f) Cowan LD, and oth-
    ers. Cancer mortality and lipid and lipoprotein levels. The Lipid Re-
    search Clinics' program mortality follow-up study. *American Journal
    of Epidemiology* 131, 468-482, 1990.
2. Feinleib M. Summary of a workshop on cholesterol and
    noncardiovascular disease mortality. *Preventive Medicine* 11, 360-367,
    1982.
3. In many studies the risk of developing cancer with low blood chole-
    sterol levels was just as great as the risk of developing coronary heart
    disease with high levels.
4. To learn more about free radicals, read: Halliwell B, Gutteridge JMC.
    Free Radicals in Biology and Medicine. Clarendon Press, Oxford 1989
    (2nd ed.)
5. The harmful effects of polyunsaturated fatty acids are described in the
    following papers. More references are found in the papers. (a) Harman
    D. Atherosclerosis: possible ill-effects of the use of highly unsaturated
    fats to lower serum-cholesterol levels. *The Lancet* 2, 1116-1117, 1957;
    (b) Pinckney ER. The potential toxicity of excessive polyunsaturates.
    Do not let the patient harm himself. *American Heart Journal* 85, 723-
    726, 1973; (c) Editorial. Are PUFA harmful? *British Medical Journal*
    4, 1-2, 1973; (d) West CE, Redgrave TG. Reservations on the use of
    polyunsaturated fats in human nutrition. *Search* 5, 90-96, 1974; (e)
    Vitale JJ, Broitman SA. Lipids and immune function. *Cancer Research*
    41, 3706-3710, 1981; (f) Bennett M, Uauy R, Grundy SM. Dietary fatty
    acid effects on T-cell-mediated immunity in mice infected with Myco-
    plasma pulmonis or given carcinogens by injection. *American Journal
    of Pathology* 126, 103-113, 1987; (g) Racker E. Calories don't count if
    you don't use them. *American Journal of Medicine* 35, 143-144, 1963.
6. McHugh MI and others. Immunosuppression with polyunsaturated fatty
    acids in renal transplantation. *Transplantation* 24, 263-267, 1977.
7. Alexander JC, Valli VE, Chanin BE. Biological observations from feed-
    ing heated corn oil and heated peanut oil to rats. *Journal of Toxicology
    and Environmental Health* 21, 295-309, 1987
8. Richie J and others. Edema and hemolytic anemia in premature in-

fants. *New England Journal of Medicine* 279, 1185-1190, 1968
9. Dam H, Söndergaard E. The encephalomalacia producing effect of arachidonic and linoleic acids. *Zeitschrift für Ernährungswissenschaft* 2, 217-222, 1962.
10. Editorial. Atherosclerosis and auto-oxidation of cholesterol. *The Lancet* 1, 964-965, 1980. Steinberg D and others. Beyond cholesterol. Modifications of low-density lipoprotein that increases its atherogenicity. *New England Journal of Medicine* 320, 915-924, 1989.
11. Watanabe rabbits have the same hereditary metabolic defect as individuals with familial hypercholesterolemia and develop very high blood cholesterol levels on their usual vegetarian diet.
12. Carew TE, Schwenke DC, Steinberg D. Antiatherogenic effect of probucol unrelated to its hypocholesterolemic effect. *Proceedings of the National Academy of Science* USA 84, 7725-7729, 1987. Blood cholesterol of the control rabbits was lowered with another cholesterol-lowering drug, lovastatin which has no antioxidant effect. But it was the number of fatty streaks that decreased, not the degree of atherosclerosis.
13. Clubb FJ and others. Effect of dietary omega-3 fatty acid on serum lipids, plasma function and atherosclerosis in Watanabe heritable hyperlipidemic rabbits. *Atherosclerosis* 9, 529-537, 1989.
14. Scott Grundy, the main designer of the dietary recommendations from the National Heart, Lung and Blood Institute, wrote that it is not a good idea to substitute fatty acids of animal origin with polyunsaturated fatty acids: high intakes. . . might not be entirely safe. Of special concern to Grundy is that high intakes of linoleic acid (the most prevalent poyunsaturated fatty acid) may promote cancer in human beings as it does in laboratory animals. Besides, he gave most of the arguments I presented in Chapter 7, and he concluded that intakes above 7 percent of total calories seemingly cannot be advocated with prudence. Grundy did not explain how he found the limit of just 7 percent, and his warnings against polyunsaturated fat appeared in the middle of a large review article concerning something else, and nothing was mentioned about it in the summary of his paper (Grundy SM. Multifactorial etiology of hypercholesterolemia. Implications for prevention of coronary heart disease. *Circulation* 86, 1619-1635, 1992).
15. A thorough review of the history, chemistry and biological effects of the *trans* fatty acids is found in Enig MG. *Trans fatty acids in the food supply: a comprehensive report covering 60 years of research.* Enig Associates, Inc., Silver Spring, MD, 1993.
16. Hanis T and others. Effects of dietary *trans*-fatty acids on reproductive performance of Wistar rats. *British Journal of Nutrition* 61, 519-529, 1989.
17. Teter BB, Sampugna J, Keeny M. Milk fat depression in C57Bl/6J mice consuming partially hydrogenated fat. *Journal of Nutrition* 120, 818-824, 1990.
18. Koletzko B. *Trans* fatty acids may impair biosynthesis of long-chain polyunsaturates and growth in man. *Acta Pediatrica* 81, 302-306, 1992.
19. Atal S and others. Comparison of body weight and adipose tissue in

male C57Bl/6J mice fed diets with and without *trans* fatty acids. *Lipids* 29, 319-325, 1994

20. Mensick RP and Katan MB. Effect of dietary *trans* fatty acids on high-density and low-density lipoprotein cholesterol levels in healthy subjects. *New England Journal of Medicine* 323, 439-445, 1990.
21. Muldoon MF, Manuck SB, Matthews KA. Lowering cholesterol concentrations and mortality: a quantitative review of primary prevention trials. *British Medical Journal* 301, 309-314, 1990.
22. Horrobin DF. Lowering cholesterol concentrations and mortality. *British Medical Journal* 301, 554, 1990.
23. Lindberg G and others. Low serum cholesterol concentration and short term mortality from injuries in men and women. *British Medical Journal* 305, 277-279, 1992.
24. Golomb BA. Cholesterol and violence: is there a connection? *Annals of Internal Medicine* 128, 478-487, 1998.
25. Iso H and others. Serum cholesterol levels and six-year mortality from stroke in 350,977 men screened for the multiple risk factor intervention trial. *New England Journal of Medicine* 320, 904-910, 1989.

Chapter 8

1. Consensus Conference: Lowering blood cholesterol to prevent heart disease. *Journal of the American Medical Association* 253, 2080-2086, 1985. The description of the conference is mainly based on Thomas J. Moore. *Heart Failure*, Random House, New York, 1989. Moore's book is a critical portrayal of the buildup to the cholesterol campaign. His views have been violently criticized by the diet-heart proponents. However, no one has questioned his description of the conference.
2. According to Moore, the *Report and Conclusions* had been written before the meeting.
3. Some of the many critical voices are listed here: (a) Palumbo PJ. National cholesterol education program: does the emperor have any clothes? *Mayo Clinic Proceedings* 63, 88-90, 1988; (b) Oliver MF. Consensus or nonsensus conferences on coronary heart disease. *The Lancet* 1, 1087-1089, 1985; (c) Merz B. Low-fat diet may be imprudent for some, say opponents of population-based cholesterol control. *Journal of the American Medical Association* 256, 2779-2780, 1986; (d) Pinckney ER, Smith RL. Statistical analysis of lipid research clinic's program. *The Lancet* 1, 503, 1987. Pinckney and Smith conclude that the US government via the NHLBI has launched a nationwide program to alter the diet of Americans, based on a study (costing $150 million of public money) that had a faulty statistical analysis. What is more, the statistical defects were known to the trial's organisers and to the journal that published the results. Patel C; (e) The lipid research clinic's trial. *The Lancet* 1, 633-634, 1984. Patel has calculated that if the result of the LRC trial is transferred to England and Wales, one of every 400 coronary deaths could be saved each year, amounting to the cost of about 140 million pounds a year and of gastrointestinal side effects in more

than 130,000 healthy individuals; (f) Editorial. *The Lancet* 1, 333-334, 1988. The author stressed the fact that there is little correlation between dietary fat intake and cholesterol level, that no convincing dietary prevention study had been published, and that the increase in deaths from other causes in the drug trials cannot be ignored simply because it did not form part of the hypothesis that these trials were designed to test.

Chapter 9

1. Enig MG. *Trans fatty acids in the food supply: a comprehensive report covering 60 years of research.* Enig Associates, Silver Spring, MD, 1993.
2. Enig MG. *Know Your Fats: The Complete Primer for Understanding the Nutrition of Fats, Oils, and Cholesterol.* Bethesda Press, Silver Spring, MD, 2000.
3. Gurr MI. Dietary lipids and coronary heart disease: old evidence, new perspective. *Progress of Lipid Research* 31, 195-243, 1992.
4. Mann GV. Diet-heart: end of an era. *New England Journal of Medicine* 297, 644-650, 1977.
5. Mann GV. Coronary heart disease: "Doing the wrong things." *Nutrition Today* July/August, p. 12-14, 1985.
6. Oliver MF. Dietary fat and coronary heart disease. *British Heart Journal* 58, 423-428, 1987.
7. Oliver MF. Might treatment of hypercholesterolaemia increase non-cardiac mortality? *The Lancet* 337, 1529-1531, 1991. Other critical papers by Oliver: (a) Oliver MF. Consensus or nonsensus conferences on coronary heart disease. *The Lancet* 1, 1087-1089, 1985; (b) Oliver MF. Dietary fat and coronary heart disease. *British Heart Journal* 58, 423-428, 1987; (c) Oliver MF. Reducing cholesterol does not reduce mortality. Journal of the *American College of Cardiology* 12, 814-7, 1988; (d) Oliver MF. Doubts about preventing coronary heart disease. Multiple interventions in middle-aged men may do more harm than good. *British Medical Journal* 304, 393-394, 1992; (e) Oliver MF. National cholesterol policies. *European Heart Journal* 14, 581-583, 1993.
8. Pinckney ER and Pinckney C. *The Cholesterol Controversy.* Sherbourne Press, Los Angeles, 1973.
9. Reiser R. Saturated fat in the diet and serum cholesterol concentration: a critical examination of the literature. *American Journal of Clinical Nutrition* 26, 524-555, 1973.
10. Reiser R. A commentary on the rationale of the diet-heart statement of the American Heart Association. *American Journal of Clinical Nutrition* 40, 654-658, 1984.
11. Professor Rosch's views on the cholesterol issue are published in *Health and Stress. The Newsletter of The American Institute of Stress,* 1995, number 1; 1998, number 1; 1999, number 8; 2001, numbers 2,4,7. See also Rosch, PJ. Statins don't work by lowering lipids. Electronic response in *British Medical Journal* 2001,17. Nov and Rosch PJ. Com-

ment to: Guidelines for Diagnosis and Treatment of High Cholesterol. *Journal of the American Medical Association* 286, 2001, 2400. (Read also four other letters and Scott Grundy's "non-answer.")

12. Friedman M, Rosenman RH, Byers SO. Deranged cholesterol metabolism and its possible relationship to human atherosclerosis: a review. *Journal of Gerontology* 10, 60-85, 1955. Rosenman RH. The questionable roles of the diet and serum cholesterol in the incidence of ischemic heart disease and its 20th century changes. *Homeostasis* 34, 1-43, 1993.

13. Smith RL. *Diet, blood cholesterol and coronary heart disease: a critical review of the literature.* Vector Enterprises. Vol. 1, 1989; Vol. 2, 1991. The two books above are indispensable for those who are interested in the diet-heart idea.

14. *The Cholesterol Conspiracy.* Warren H. Green, Inc. St. Louis, 1991. A somewhat more popular edition, but still exhaustive of Dr. Smith's study, listed above. A short summary of Russell Smith's criticism is published in Dietary lipids and heart disease. The contriving of a relationship. *American Clinical Laboratory* November, p. 26-33, 1989.

15. Stehbens WE. An appraisal of the epidemic rise of coronary heart disease and its decline. *The Lancet* 1, 606-611, 1987. Stehbens WE. The lipid hypothesis and the role of hemodynamics in atherogenesis. *Progress in Cardiovascular Diseases.* 33, 119-136, 1990.

16. (a) Werkö L. Risk factors and coronary heart disease—facts or fancy? *American Heart Journal* 91, 87-98, 1976; (b) Werkö L. Prevention of heart attacks. *Annals of Clinical Research* 11, 71-79, 1979, (c) Werkö L. Diet, lipids and heart attacks. *Acta Medica Scandinavica* 206, 435-439, 1979; (d) Werkö L. The enigma of coronary heart disease and its prevention. *Acta Medica Scandinavica* 221, 323-333, 1987; (e) Werkö L. Analysis of the MRFIT screenees: a methodological study. *Journal of Internal Medicine* 237, 507-518, 1995.

17. (a) Altschule MD. The cholesterol problem. *Medical Counterpoint* January, p. 11, 1970; Can diet prevent atherogenesis? If so, what diet? *Medical Counterpoint* November, p. 13, 1970;
(b) Meade TW, Chakrabarti R. Arterial disease research: observation or intervention? *The Lancet* 2, 913-916, 1972;
(c) McMichael J. Prevention of coronary heart-disease. *The Lancet* 2, 569, 1976;
(d) Mohler H. Die Cholesterin-Neurose. Der Standpunkt des Ernährungswissenschafters. *Salle-Sauerländer,* Frankfurt am Main 1978;
(e) McMichael J. Fats and arterial disease. *American Heart Journal* 98, 409-412, 1979;
(f) Ahrens EH. Dietary fats and coronary heart disease: unfinished business. *The Lancet* 2, 1345-1348, 1979;
(g) Stallones RA. Ischemic heart disease and lipids in blood and diet. *Annual Reviews of Nutrition* 3, 155-185, 1983;
(h) Ahrens EH. The diet-heart question in 1985: has it really been settled? *The Lancet* 1, 1085-1087, 1985;

(i) American Academy of Pediatrics Committee on Nutrition. Prudent life-style for children: dietary fat and cholesterol. *Pediatrics* 78, 521-5. 1986;

(j) Cliff WJ. Coronary heart disease: Animal fat on trial. *Pathology* 19, 325-328, 1987;

(k) McCormick J, Skrabanek P. Coronary heart disease is not preventable by population interventions. *The Lancet* 2, 839-41, 1988;

(l) McGee CT. Heart Frauds. Uncovering the Biggest Health Scam in History. HealthWise, Colorado Springs 2001;

(m) Skrabanek P, McCormick J. *Follies and Fallacies in Medicine*. Tarragon Press, Glasgow, 1989; Skrabanek P. Nonsensus consensus. *The Lancet* 335, 1446-1447, 1990;

(n) Moore TJ. *Heart Failure*. Random House, New York, 1989;

(o) Hulley SB, Walsh JMB, Newman TB. Health policy on blood cholesterol. Time to change directions. *Circulation* 86, 1026-1029, 1992;

(p) Smith G Davey, Pekkanen J. Should there be a moratorium on the use of cholesterol lowering drugs? *British Medical Journal* 304, 431-434, 1992;

(q) Berger M. The cholesterol non-consensus. In: Somogyi JC, Biró G, Hötzel D (eds): *Nutrition and Cardiovascular Risks*. Bibliotheca Nutritio et Dieta nr 49, 125-130, 1992;

(r) Berger M. Der Cholesterin-Non-Konsensus in der Primärprävention der koronaren Herzkrankheit. *Zeitschrift für Kardiologie* 82, 399-405, 1993;

(s) Apfelbaum M. *Vivre avec du cholesterol*. Editions du Rocher, Monaco 1992;

(t) Sieber R. Cholesterol removal from animal food—can it be justified? *Lebensmittel-Wissenschaft und Technologie* 26, 375-387, 1993;

(u) Olson RE. CHD intervention trials and all-cause mortality. *Circulation* 90, 2569-2570, 1994;

(v) Atrens DM. The questionable wisdom of a low-fat diet and cholesterol reduction. *Social Science and Medicine* 39, 433-447, 1994;

(w) Texon, M. *Hemodynamic basis of atherosclerosis with critique of the cholesterol-heart disease hypothesis*. Begell House, New York 1995;

(x) Worm N. Ernährung und koronare Herzkrankheit: Wie sinnvoll ist diät? *Versicherungsmedizin* 47, 116-121, 1995.

Index

About the Author

Uffe Ravnskov was born 1934 in Copenhagen, Denmark. He received his medical degree from the University of Copenhagen in 1961. During the next seven years, he worked at various surgical, roentgenological, neurological, pediatric and medical departments in Denmark and Sweden. He then began scientific studies at the Departments of Nephrology and Clinical Chemistry at the University Hospital in Lund, Sweden, and was awarded his Ph.D. in 1973.

Dr. Ravnskov entered private practice as a specialist in internal medicine and nephrology in 1979 and since that time has worked as a family doctor and independent researcher in Lund.

Since 1990 he has published more than 50 critical papers and letters about the alleged association between cholesterol and cardiovascular disease in well-known Scandinavian and international peer-reviewed medical journals. In 1999, he received the Skrabanek Award given by Trinity College of Dublin, Ireland for original contributions in the field of medical skepticism. Dr. Ravnskov has also published many critical articles on this subject in major Scandinavian newspapers and is a member of the expert panel of the *Journal of the Swedish Medical Association* (Läkartidningen) and *Tidskriften Medikament*, a Swedish medical journal.

Among his many other scientific contributions are more than 20 papers on the cause of glomerulonephritis, which in most countries is the most common cause of end-stage kidney failure.

His book *The Cholesterol Myth* was published in Sweden 1991 and in Finland a year later. His website on the subject, (www.ravnskov.nu/cholesterol.htm), posted in 1997, has generated intense interest. *The Cholesterol Myths* is an updated and expanded version of the website and his earlier book.

Books About Diet and Health from NewTrends Publishing

Nourishing Traditions
The Cookbook that Challenges
Politically Correct Nutrition and the Diet Dictocrats
by Sally Fallon
with Mary G. Enig, PhD

For those no longer afraid of saturated fat and cholesterol, here is the book that delineates the health advantages of traditional foods, including meat, butter, eggs and whole-milk products. Includes important information on preparation of grains and legumes, nourishing bone broths, and diets for growing children. Contains more than 700 recipes and a wealth of information on diet and health. Quality paperback. 688 pages. $25.

The Fourfold Path to Healing
Working with the Laws of
Nutrition, Therapeutics, Movement and Meditation
in the Art of Medicine
by Thomas Cowan, MD
with Sally Fallon and Jaimen McMillan

A holistic approach to modern diseases, including proper diet, modern and ancient therapies, corrective movement and thoughtful meditation. Dr. Cowan's approach is at once poetic and practical, uniting all that is best of the modern and traditional healing paradigms. To be published Fall 2002. Quality paperback. $25.

Toll Free Order Line 877-707-1776
Or online ordering at www.NewTrendsPublishing.com

Cholesterol Conversion Table

mg/dl (Used in the US)	mmol/L (Used in Europe)
120	3.1
140	3.6
160	4.1
180	4.6
200	5.1
220	5.6
240	6.2
260	6.7
280	7.2
300	7.7
320	8.2
340	8.7
360	9.2
380	9.7
400	10.3
500	12.8
600	15.4
700	17.9
800	20.5
900	23.1
1000	25.6